Managing Childhood Anxiety

by Natasha Burgert, MD, FAAP

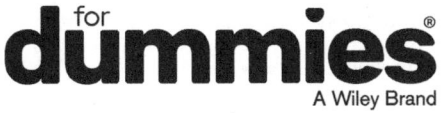

A Wiley Brand

Managing Childhood Anxiety For Dummies®

Published by: **John Wiley & Sons, Inc.**, 111 River Street, Hoboken, NJ 07030-5774, www.wiley.com

For general information on our other products and services, please contact our Customer Care Department within the U.S. at 877-762-2974, outside the U.S. at 317-572-3993, or fax 317-572-4002. For technical support, please visit https://hub.wiley.com/community/support/dummies.

Wiley publishes in a variety of print and electronic formats and by print-on-demand. Some material included with standard print versions of this book may not be included in e-books or in print-on-demand. If this book refers to media that is not included in the version you purchased, you may download this material at http://booksupport.wiley.com. For more information about Wiley products, visit www.wiley.com.

Library of Congress Control Number is available from the publisher.

ISBN 978-1-394-32955-7 (pbk); ISBN 978-1-394-32957-1 (ebk); ISBN 978-1-394-32956-4 (ebk)

Printed and bound by CPI Group (UK) Ltd, Croydon, CR0 4YY

C9781394329557_270625

Table of Contents

Introduction

Let me guess why you picked up this book. Maybe you think your child is worrying too much, and you're not sure if that's normal. At a recent doctor's appointment, did the doctor suggest your child's abdominal pain or headache is from anxiety — and you're not sure whether you believe it? Or are you one of the millions of parents caring for a young child who was recently diagnosed with an anxiety disorder, and you're looking for all the help you can get?

No matter the reason, I'm glad that you are here. I wrote this book for you.

Millions of families all over the world are looking for ways to manage childhood anxiety. Anxiety is one of the most commonly diagnosed mental health conditions in young children today. According to 2021 data from the Centers for Disease Control, 11.3 percent of children ages 5 to 11 years old received mental health treatment in the past 12 months. Just like you, the parents of these kids are looking for ways to effectively help their children learn to live and thrive with anxiety. This book is the road map you need.

About This Book

Managing Childhood Anxiety For Dummies is designed to help parents of children ages 4–11 through the process of anxiety diagnosis and treatment. In these pages, you find a strong foundation of education, understanding, and support. What makes this book unique is that it's written from the perspective of an experienced, board-certified pediatrician who has spent the last 20 years caring for hundreds of families just like yours. That's me.

This book is filled with what I want my patient families to know about childhood anxiety. It's everything I wish I had time to say when a parent asks, "Dr. Natasha, I think she may have anxiety. Where do I start?" — without the constraints of a 20-minute office visit.

Of course, this book doesn't replace the guidance and care given to you by your child's healthcare provider. However, it will help you walk into their office prepared to ask smart questions and with a clearer sense of what you hope to achieve.

A quick note: Sidebars (shaded boxes of text) dig into the details of a given topic related to childhood anxiety, but they aren't crucial to understanding it. Feel free to read them or skip them. You can pass over the text accompanied by the Technical Stuff icon, too. The text marked with this icon gives some interesting but nonessential information about managing anxiety.

One last thing: Within this book, you may note that some web addresses break across two lines of text. If you're reading this book in print and want to visit one of these web pages, simply key in the web address exactly as it's noted in the text, pretending as though the line break doesn't exist. If you're reading this as an e-book, you've got it easy — just click the web address to be taken directly to the web page.

Foolish Assumptions

As an experienced pediatrician, I understand that there are all types of families. Within these families are dynamic, kind, resilient, smart, talented kids who are deeply loved. I assume you are a parent to one of these amazing kids, and you'd do anything in your power to keep them safe and well.

I also assume that you're busy, stressed, a little burned out, and trying to figure out what you're going to make for dinner in the next 20 minutes. That being said, I'm going to get you to the bottom line quickly. I include explanations only where I think they're important, and I add references if you want to go deeper on your own time.

Icons Used in This Book

Like all *For Dummies* books, this book features icons to help you navigate the information. Here's what they mean.

REMEMBER

This icon indicates summaries of key concepts, and many are repeated throughout the book. If you don't remember anything else, you'll want to remember these.

TIP

To highlight action steps and tools that you can use to help manage your child's anxiety, I use this icon.

TECHNICAL STUFF

I put this icon next to science-y information that I think is cool but not necessary for you to understand the elements of a given section or chapter.

WARNING

This icon calls out things that are exceptionally dangerous or important for your child's health and safety.

Beyond the Book

There's more than the advice in these analog or digital pages. In addition to the information and guidance on child anxiety that I offer here, there's more on dummies.com. Find this book's Cheat Sheet at wwww.dummies.com and search for "Managing Childhood Anxiety For Dummies Cheat Sheet." There you find information about types of childhood anxiety, how to put together a calming kit for an anxious kid, and more.

Where to Go from Here

You can read this book from cover to cover, and I hope you do! But under the assumption that your time is limited, feel free to jump to the chapter you need the most today. Looking for a therapist, but don't know what all the letters mean? Jump to

Chapter 9. Did your child's doctor suggest anxiety medication, and that's freaking you out? Find my take in Chapter 10. Maybe you need help with screen time or nutrition advice. That's in Chapter 13.

Regardless of where you start, I hope you find value within these pages. I hope it offers what you're looking for and becomes something you reference in the future. Most importantly, I hope this book shines light on the amazing person your child is today, while also acknowledging your dedication, effort, and unyielding love that is guiding them into their future. Let's get started.

1

Getting Started with Managing Childhood Anxiety

Find out how children are different biologically, developmentally, and emotionally from adults. Explore how these physical differences in brain form and function create natural periods of higher emotional responsiveness, which evolve over time.

Acknowledge and respect the vast number of kids and parents who struggle with anxiety. Evaluate current anxiety statistics and underlying factors that contribute to developing anxiety, making it clear that families aren't alone. Move toward a path of acceptance and readiness to lovingly support a child through their anxiety experience.

Walk through normal child development to discover a framework critical to understanding how anxiety presents in children, including what common symptoms and behaviors of anxiety look like in kids. Distinguish normal from abnormal behaviors and see that young children don't talk about their anxiety; they show it.

Recognize that child anxiety symptoms can include physical symptoms like stomachaches, headaches, and sleep changes. Discover ways to support a child at home with physical complaints, and look for red flags that should make parents concerned. In addition, find medical conditions that may mimic childhood anxiety.

Chapter **1**

Worrying About Your Child's Worries

nxiety is a protector and defender. Without it, we wouldn't be able to survive or properly care for the ones we love. But when feelings of worry and fear become irrational, all-consuming, or cause us to change our behavior, that's when anxiety becomes unhealthy and no longer performs its desired function.

In this chapter, you discover some anxiety basics, including why childhood anxiety is particularly unique. You start to think about anxiety as a medical diagnosis. Finally, you see that childhood anxiety is exceptionally treatable, and treatment starts with you.

Defining Anxiety

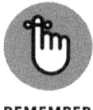

REMEMBER

Childhood anxiety represents a spectrum of emotional, behavioral, and physical responses characterized by persistent worry, fear, and apprehension that exceeds developmental norms and interferes with daily functioning.

As a pediatrician, I regularly see how anxiety uniquely manifests in children through physical complaints like stomachaches or headaches, behavioral changes such as school avoidance or tantrums, and cognitive patterns involving excessive worry. When these symptoms get big enough to pull kids away from the things they need or love to do, I become concerned that a child may be suffering from an anxiety disorder.

The importance of addressing childhood anxiety cannot be overstated. Longitudinal studies show that children with untreated anxiety are more likely to develop depression, substance use disorders, and even more severe anxiety conditions later in life. Beyond these long-term concerns, childhood anxiety immediately impacts academic performance, social development, family functioning, and overall quality of life.

TIP

There are ways to reduce the impact of anxiety's long-term effects. This book walks you through these evidence-supported interventions, including many things you can do at home. See Parts 3 and 4.

Analyzing Anxiety

Childhood anxiety is on the rise. In fact, doctor visits for anxiety have increased from 1.4 percent in 2006 to 4.2 percent in 2018. In my private practice, I see one or two children per day for anxiety management. Multiply that by the 67,000 pediatricians in the United States alone, and you can appreciate how common anxiety disorders are in today's youth.

Seeing rising rates of anxiety

Researchers are devoting countless hours of expertise to determine why rates of child anxiety are on the rise. Theories include increased public awareness, pandemic fallout, and social media use. See Chapter 3.

REMEMBER

Regardless of the cause of anxiety's rise, the message is clear: Kids are more anxious than ever before. Every child, including yours, deserves to be heard, seen, and supported if they show signs of worry and stress. Being aware of anxiety and its symptoms is the first step.

Finding the roots of anxiety

Childhood anxiety results from a blend of biological and environmental factors. Biological factors are determined by your child's genetics, temperament, and brain development. Environmental factors refer to elements or conditions in a child's surroundings that influence their health. You find these factors discussed in various ways throughout this book. Also, you find ways to modify or impact factors you think are triggering your child's anxiety symptoms.

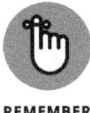

REMEMBER

Although you cannot take anxiety away from your child, you can change the intensity and duration of their anxiety experience.

Looking for Anxiety in Children

One of the biggest challenges — and joys — of working with kids is that they are physiologically and developmentally different than adults. These inherent differences make identifying, evaluating, and diagnosing anxiety in young kids difficult.

Appreciating child development

When working with kids, it's important to take a child's developmental phase into account. As children grow, they pass through expected phases while acquiring increasingly complex skills, called *developmental milestones.* Milestone progress from infancy through young adulthood is predictable in sequence, with one skill building upon another.

TIP

If you're looking for a comprehensive list of childhood developmental milestones, the CDC has a free, interactive app called "CDC's Milestone Tracker." Find additional online resources in the Appendix.

At every well-child visit, pediatricians assess social-emotional milestones. These key developmental achievements (found in Chapter 2) involve a child's ability to understand emotions, form relationships, express feelings, and navigate social interactions in age-appropriate ways. Social-emotional milestones are especially important to assess for kids struggling with fear and worry.

TIP

If you are unsure whether your child's behavior is normal, call your child's pediatrician. We get questions from worried parents every day and can let you know if additional evaluation is needed.

Showing, not telling

When you're frightened, your body surges with stress hormones, all aimed at one goal — to protect. This hormone cascade prepares your body to fight, run away, or hide from a threat. This happens in kids too, but they lack the language to express what their brain and body are feeling. Instead of using words, kids *show* anxiety though behaviors.

Anxiety's uncomfortable symptoms lead to *avoidance behaviors* — a key characteristic in all types of childhood anxiety. Avoidance behaviors are actions kids take to escape or prevent anxiety-provoking situations. If avoidance behaviors are allowed to continue, the connection is reinforced in their brain as an effective way to avoid danger and fear, becoming a learned behavior over time.

REMEMBER

Kids don't tell you they are feeling anxious, they show you through changes in their behavior.

Checking out various anxiety types

If a child's anxiety behaviors are not age-appropriate, or if they are interfering with the things the child loves to play and do, that's when professionals consider the possibility of an anxiety disorder. In young children, some anxiety disorder types are more common than others. For details of the most common anxiety disorders in young children, including separation anxiety disorder, social anxiety disorder, generalized anxiety disorder, and specific phobias see Chapter 4.

Getting the Diagnosis

Diagnosing a childhood anxiety disorder requires specialized assessments that consider development, cognition, and family involvement. The good news is that decades of research have focused on child anxiety identification and treatment. Today, there are evidence-supported interventions to help identify kids more quickly and guide treatment in age-appropriate ways.

Starting with your child's doctor

An anxiety diagnosis starts with a trip to your child's healthcare provider. During the appointment, you can share your child's story and why you're worried about anxiety. In turn, your child's doctor will evaluate them for any medical conditions that may be contributing to their symptoms. The doctor can also find ways to support the physical symptoms of anxiety your child may be experiencing. For more on doctors' visits see Chapter 7.

TIP

Not all child health providers evaluate children for anxiety. Talk with your child's doctor to find out whether they handle mental health concerns or suggest going elsewhere for an assessment.

Considering alternative diagnoses

If an anxiety disorder is suspected, or if your child's behaviors are unclear, tapping into the expertise of a child psychologist can be helpful. During a comprehensive psychological evaluation, your observations of your child's behaviors will be considered, in addition to information directly gathered from your child.

Some different diagnoses that psychologists consider when evaluating a child with anxiety behaviors include the following (see Chapter 8):

>> Attention-deficit/hyperactivity disorder (ADHD)

>> Oppositional defiant disorder (ODD)

>> Learning challenges

>> Sensory processing disorder (SPD)

>> Autism spectrum disorder (ASD)

TECHNICAL STUFF

Up to half of children with an anxiety disorder have an additional health condition or disorder, referred to as a *co-morbidity.* Having more than one diagnosis can create interactions that may complicate diagnosis, treatment, and management.

Accepting your child's anxiety

When a child is diagnosed with an anxiety disorder, families often feel overwhelmed. It's tough to see your child struggle, and guilt or shame may arise. I encourage you to let go of these feelings — they're not yours to hold. The sooner you release them, the sooner you can confidently support your child and work toward symptom remission.

REMEMBER

Your child with anxiety is not broken, and there's nothing to "fix." Anxiety is a part of who they are and always will be. It's another aspect of your child you're learning about as they grow, offering you more ways to show love, support, and care.

Exploring Treatment

In recent decades, there have been significant advancements in child neuropsychology. Clinical research findings have led to more accurate and consistent diagnostic tools. In addition, advancements in brain imaging and neurobiological research have discovered ways to bring anxiety symptoms into remission.

A comprehensive anxiety management plan includes a variety of components, depending on the level of support a child requires. Parts of the medical plan may include all or some of the following.

Leaning into therapy

Cognitive behavioral therapy (CBT) is the gold standard treatment for childhood anxiety. Modern psychological therapies are also being used to treat anxiety in children. Chapter 9 explores these options in detail.

TIP

Therapy isn't just for kids with diagnosed anxiety disorders. Children can benefit from talking with a therapist during times of transition, for emotional guidance, working through trauma or grief, or whenever emotions or behaviors start interfering with daily life.

Fueling the anxious brain

Kids need fuel to grow healthy brains and bodies, and a variety of nutritional factors are required for this work. But kids with anxiety disorders often have unique eating habits that make it more difficult to get these essential nutrients. With your doctor's guidance, nutritional deficits can be identified and supported as part of an anxiety plan.

Providing protection

Part 4 of this book is dedicated to many things that buffer anxiety's negative effects. These things promote healthy emotional learning, self-regulation, and relationship building. Additionally, things like sleep, nutrition, and exercise decrease the physical effects of chronic stress, leading to increased resilience and stress reduction.

Your child is unique; their anxiety is not. For all kids with anxiety, treatment plans focus on modifying the well-known biochemical and developmental pathways that reinforce fear behaviors.

Considering anxiety medications

For some children, anxiety symptoms interfere so significantly in their daily lives that therapy alone isn't enough. Additionally, some kids are unable or unwilling to particulate in therapy. In situations like these, adding medication to an anxiety plan is medically necessary to bring their symptoms into remission.

The suggestion of an anxiety medication can make parents uneasy. In my experience, much of this apprehension is founded in personal experience, family anecdotes, concerning social media posts, or frank misinformation. Straight talk on anxiety medications is found in Chapter 10.

Anxiety treatment sometimes requires using medications to boost natural hormones and neurotransmitters. Most of these medications focus on increasing the bioavailability of serotonin — 90 percent of which is found in the gut!

Finding support at school

Kids spend most of their waking hours at school. For kids with anxiety, having dedicated plans to ensure adequate support should be part of their educational experience. These plans can include anything from allowing a child with anxiety-triggered abdominal pain to visit the school counselor during the day, all the way to creating comprehensive support plans like an Individualized Educational Plan (IEP). See Chapter 14 for more information on thriving in school.

Prioritizing safety

Although sobering and upsetting, it's important to recognize that kids with anxiety are at increased risk of death by suicide, and the average age of suicide death is declining. Being aware of actions you can take to decrease a child's risk of suicide is imperative when caring for any child. Don't miss this valuable information in Chapter 10.

Helping Your Child Where You Can

One of the hardest parts of parenting is even when you try your all, you ultimately don't have control of your child's future. In spite of this sobering truth, you're essential to supporting your child's anxiety experience. This starts with managing your own emotional regulation and mental health. See Chapter 12 for details.

Beginning with you

One of the biggest things that influences your child's experience with anxiety is *you*. Taking care of your own mental health isn't a luxury — it's a necessity. Kids are incredibly attuned to their caregivers, and if you're overwhelmed, stressed, or emotionally drained, it becomes much harder to provide the calm, steady support they need.

If you're struggling with anxiety, depression, grief, or other emotional stress, it affects how you parent, disrupts your ability to support your child, and raises the risk of long-term mental health challenges in your family. When you prioritize your own well-being — through therapy, self-care, or simply making time to recharge — you equip yourself to show up as the best version of yourself for your child.

REMEMBER

Being mentally healthy does not mean being happy. It means having emotions that are appropriate for the moment and managing those emotions well.

Seeing it through

Your child needs you. They need you to show them what mental wellness and healthy emotional regulation look like. They need you to be objective and clear. They need you to get them the support they need today, the next day, and the next.

I know this isn't easy. Supporting your child with anxiety may be exceptionally challenging for you right now because of your own personal health history, the current relationship with your child, or another significant barrier. But I also know taking one small step forward can reveal a path you may not be able to see from where you are standing. Together, we move ahead.

Chapter **2**

Recognizing That Kids Aren't Little Adults

On the first day of pediatric residency training, doctors are taught the pediatrician's "golden rule": Kids aren't little adults. Throughout this book, I hope to convince you of this truth. Children are growing, shape-shifting individuals whose biology and physiology are different from grown adults. Learning about and respecting these differences is one way you can better understand and love your child for who they are today.

If you are struggling to make sense of your child's emotions and behavior, digging deeper into basic childhood development can be eye-opening. Many parents overestimate their child's emotional abilities at different ages, expecting more self-regulation than their brain development allows. As kids grow, their emotional regulation improves but only as fast as their brain matures. When parents misjudge this, it often leads to unchecked frustration and relational stress.

Understanding developmental phases helps you show compassion for both your child and yourself on the tough days. When you see certain behaviors, you'll have the framework to understand what your child may be experiencing or trying to communicate. Along the way, this approach can guide you in raising an emotionally mature young adult.

In this chapter, you find out about basic brain growth during early childhood. I call out relevant chemical communicators that are used by the brain and nervous system. Using this framework of basic neurobiology, I explain how emotions develop and why children are more emotionally expressive than adults. Finally, I summarize the reasons why working with pediatric mental health is challenging to physicians and parents alike.

Meeting the Boss: Your Child's Brain

Starting at the top — your child's brain — is key to discussing mental health. As your body's boss, the brain controls all the voluntary and involuntary actions of the *central nervous system* (CNS). The CNS is a communication highway, connecting the brain to the body. From the thoughts in your mind to how your organs function, the CNS is involved in nearly everything you do, think, and feel.

TECHNICAL STUFF

If you strung all the nerves in an adult human body end to end, the strand would be 45 feet long.

The brain is organized into different parts, each with a specific job. To handle all the amazing tasks it performs throughout life, the brain develops and operates in a hierarchy of complexity, which I describe in the following sections. As you grow, your brain progresses from managing basic tasks to handling more complex ones. Along the way, the connections required for advanced thinking and emotional processing are strengthened.

Your brain is not like your kid's brain. Different stages of life are directly influenced by the slow development and organization of brain functions over time. Although kids' brains have more neurons, *or brain cells,* the communication between neurons is not well organized, and some brain areas don't fully function until many years after birth.

REMEMBER

Brain development takes a long time. Mature brain connections happen slowly over many years. Taking the time to become familiar with the function of your child's brain as they grow increases your compassion and understanding for the emotional behaviors you observe in your child.

The vital hindbrain

The human brain is divided into three main sections: the hindbrain, the inner brain, and the outer brain. Interestingly, the growth and maturity of these brain parts happens in a specific order, and all brain growth starts in the hindbrain.

The hindbrain is essential for life. Think of the hindbrain as your body's behind-the-scenes control room. It controls all the body's basic functions that you don't have to think about, like keeping your heart beating and lungs breathing. It also helps with smooth body movements, so you don't fall over.

Even before you're born, the hindbrain is managing body systems. Because its job is so foundational, the hindbrain develops before any other brain parts form. This step-by-step growth ensures that basic functions are in place before developing any advanced abilities.

The emotional inner brain

Next, the inner brain begins to mature. This area is directly connected to the hindbrain and is present at birth. The inner brain includes the emotional processing part of the brain, called the *limbic system.* The limbic system is responsible for integrating our senses and processing information regarding our body's *homeostasis* — or balance.

Additionally, the limbic system holds the *amygdala* — a small but mighty brain part that is responsible for the expression of fear, aggression, and defense behaviors. The amygdala also plays a role in the formation and retrieval of emotional and fear-related memories, and it's the brain structure most implicated in pediatric anxiety disorders.

The thinking outer brain

The last part of the brain to functionally develop is the thinking brain, or *cortex.* When you envision the classic image of the brain's squiggly, rope-like surface, the cortex is what you see. It's connected to both the inner brain and hindbrain and makes up the thickest part of the brain.

The cortex is responsible for all the higher functioning that makes us human. It processes information from our five senses, helping us to interpret the world around us while keeping us safe. Complex pathways in the cortex signal our muscles to walk, write, or wave to a friend. The cortex also helps us understand words, whether reading a book or having a conversation.

Behind your forehead is a specific area of the outer brain called the *prefrontal cortex* (PFC). This area helps you make decisions, solve problems, stay focused, and control your emotions and impulses. The PFC also works with the inner brain to make memories, recognize faces, and make sense of how you're feeling. Find all the brain parts in Figure 2-1.

TECHNICAL STUFF

By the age of three, the brain's rapid growth gets it to about 90 percent of adult size, but the body is only 15 percent of adult size.

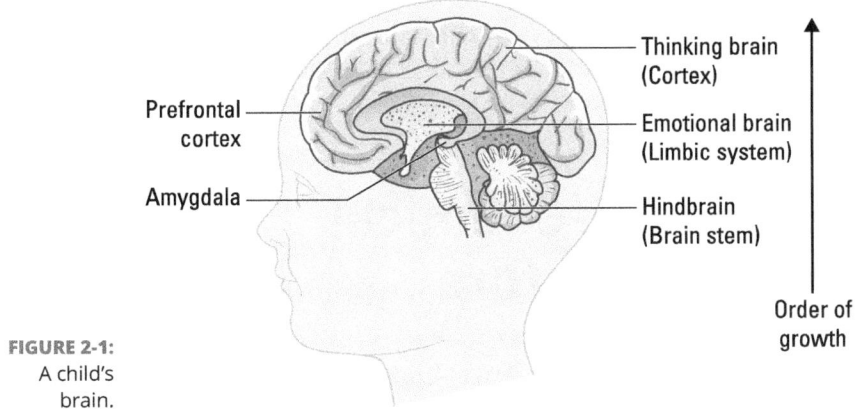

FIGURE 2-1:
A child's
brain.

© John Wiley & Sons, Inc.

Appreciating Plasticity

One of the coolest aspects of brain development is the concept of *plasticity* — or rapid periods of brain growth and learning. Think of it like this: Your brain is a super-flexible, constantly changing map. As you learn new things, gain new experiences, or even recover from injury, the brain can make new connections or re-route existing ones to help it work better.

As you age, the degree of plasticity changes. Our brain becomes less sensitive to new experiences and less likely to change or adapt. For example, by the age of three, the regulatory functions of the hindbrain are unlikely to change. However, also at the age of three, there are cortical functions that have not even begun to grow. So don't worry; old dogs *can* learn new tricks.

The cortex remains plastic throughout life, and life experiences continue to mold and change the thinking brain, no matter your age. The brain is continually creating meaningful representations of experiences and sensory information from events, allowing you to create memories — optimizing your ability to survive, adapt over time, and make many of the things that make you, *you!*

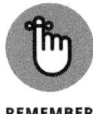

REMEMBER

In children, the quality of brain growth and connections is determined by their environment and stimulation. As a child's brain grows, it reflects the needs of the individual. In other words, children literally reflect the world in which they grow up.

Providing a loving, nurturing environment that promotes connection with caring adults is the best way to optimize the critical early years of brain growth.

Looking at Chemical Communicators

As the physical parts of the brain develop, the individual neurons communicate with each other using *neurotransmitters* — or chemical messengers. Neurotransmitters are made and released by neurons in order to carry a message to a target cell: another neuron, a muscle cell, or a gland. In the following sections, I explain how they work and describe different types.

Examining how neurotransmitters work

When a neuron wants to send a message, it releases neurotransmitters into the space between it and the target cell, called the *synapse.* Think of it like throwing a message across a gap. On the other side, the target cell receives the message when the neurotransmitter attaches to its receptor, like a key fitting into a lock. Once the neurotransmitter is attached to the receptor, the message is sent along and causes the target cell to do an action.

There are many types of neurotransmitters, each with a special job. *Excitatory* neurotransmitters are like a "green light," causing neurons to fire and spread the brain's message to nearby cells. *Inhibitory* neurotransmitters are a "red light" for brain signals, trying to slow down or stop messages from being passed along. The balance between excitatory and inhibitory neurotransmitters is important to manage the brain's signals, regulate emotions, and promote body functions.

TECHNICAL STUFF

Communication from neuron to neuron happens with insane speed. It's estimated that some neurons can transfer messages at speeds of up to 275 miles per hour. That means a pain signal from your pinky toe can reach your brain in as little as 0.01 second.

After a neurotransmitter has done its job, it becomes biologically inactive. Some neurotransmitters are recycled into the original neuron to be used again later. Other neurotransmitters are broken down by enzymes so they don't keep sending messages. Most simply drift away, lessening their ability to create any action. This process happens quickly and continuously throughout your CNS, helping everything work smoothly.

REMEMBER

An imbalance of neurotransmitters in your brain can cause problems. An overload of neurotransmitters can make the brain send too many signals. This may lead to anxiety, problems with focus or concentration, or even some types of seizures. When there is a low level of neurotransmitters, the brain does not send enough signals, possibly causing depression, difficulty moving, or trouble sleeping. The brain needs just the right amount of each neurotransmitter to keep things functioning correctly.

Meeting the messengers

Neurotransmitters are the target of many mental health medications. For more about these medications and their effect on neurotransmitters, see Chapter 10. Table 2-1 summarizes the most common chemical messengers involved in emotional development and anxiety.

TABLE 2-1 Common Neurotransmitters and Their Functions

Name and Effect	Details
Epinephrine — fight or flight	Excitatory signal that is produced in stressful situations. Increases heart rate, breathing, blood pressure, and blood sugar. Leads to physical boost and heightened awareness.
Norepinephrine — concentration	Excitatory signal that affects attention and focus, decision-making, and alertness. Also involved in the stress response. Contracts blood vessels, increasing blood pressure and heart rate.
Serotonin — mood	Inhibitory signal that regulates mood, sleep, digestion, anxiety, and pain. Can affect a large number of neurons at the same time. Influences other neurotransmitters. Too little makes you feel sad or unmotivated.

(continued)

TABLE 2-1 *(continued)*

Name and Effect	Details
Dopamine — pleasure	Both an excitatory and inhibitory signal that is wide-reaching. Plays a role in the body's reward system, helping with focus, concentration, mood, and motivation. Low levels cause slow movement, like in Parkinson's disease or depression. Increased levels can result in aggression or competitive behavior. Involved in addiction.
GABA — chill pill	Inhibitory signal that calms nerve signaling. Regulates the brain to prevent problems with concentration, sleep, and anxiety. Also contributes to motor control and vision.

Discovering How Emotions Grow

Mature emotional regulation depends on strong, two-way connections between the thinking brain (the prefrontal cortex) and the emotional brain (the amygdala). This process happens incredibly slowly in humans, with the prefrontal cortex still maturing into adulthood. It's believed that the slow process is intentional, allowing humans to leverage an extended period of plasticity.

In an adult, a mature prefrontal cortex can consciously process an emotion and refine the emotional response before the emotion is expressed. In this way, communication between the prefrontal cortex and amygdala results in more tempered and organized emotional expression. Kids, however, don't have this brain connection.

Because the emotional brain matures first, kids are less able to use the cortex to regulate their emotions. Emotional signaling arrives intensely and unfiltered into the amygdala, resulting in a more emotionally charged response. Throughout childhood, the slow maturation of the cortex-to-amygdala pathway creates a neurodevelopmental "tug-of-war." The amygdala usually wins.

REMEMBER

As a child's brain grows, there's a physical and chemical imbalance between your child's emotional center and their undeveloped higher brain functions. This results in emotional dominance left unchecked by the rational thinking brain.

Despite their underdeveloped emotional systems, kids can learn how to regulate their emotions. How do they do this? By watching you!

Throughout childhood, your child relies on *you* as their de facto prefrontal cortex. In times of stress or fear, your reaction provides physical and behavioral cues as to how they should be managing the same situation. This process, called *social referencing,* helps your child navigate uncertainty before they have experience and maturity within themselves.

REMEMBER

Expressing a calm demeanor not only soothes your child's stress, but it also shapes how they will perceive and handle fear in the future. When you stay cool as a cucumber, and your child mirrors that behavior, their brain lowers its amygdala activity. This not only provides your child with immediate soothing, but also makes the development of permanent fear memories less likely.

When a parent can't model calm during a time of stress, a child's stress response is escalated. In addition, a visibly scared parent signals to a child that a situation is dangerous or unmanageable, reinforcing fear. In this way, social referencing is one way to explain how anxiety can spread from parent to child. Discover other parental behaviors that may contribute to — and protect against — child anxiety in Chapter 12.

Exploring Social-Emotional Milestones

Parents and pediatricians monitor the expression of brain growth by watching for *developmental milestones,* or key skills and behaviors that most children can do at certain ages. Developmental milestones serve as a guideline to monitor a child's growth and help identify any areas of challenge or delay.

Most parents think of developmental milestones simply as a checklist of items their child needs to achieve. Starting to roll over a few weeks early or being the first of the cousins to say "mama" are points of parental pride. But when children don't reach milestones as expected, the checklist can turn into a list of frustrations and worries.

Despite being the pinnacle of parental comparison, developmental milestones are more than just a checklist. They are the physical expressions of brain growth. All the brain things — structure, parts, chemical messengers, cell signaling — need to be working and growing for a child to gain progressive skills. The order of process is predictable because of the way that the brain grows, from hindbrain to emotional brain to thinking brain.

REMEMBER

Milestones don't reflect a specific date or "goal." Developmental milestones are a sequence of predictable steps during childhood development that reflect a *range of* progress over time. As indispensable as the developmental milestones are for every parent and pediatrician — *and this is important* — hitting the benchmarks "on time" is less critical than seeing continued forward progress in a child's developmental path.

The developmental process cannot be sped up or slowed down; it takes time and happens over the years. Pediatricians watch for consistent, forward progress as a child grows, and they offer additional support to kids who need help meeting their personal growth goals. Just like milestones for walking and talking, the brain parts and pathways to understand and interpret emotions also follow a predictable path. In turn, there are observable and expected social-emotional milestones as children grow. These gains are intricately linked to cognitive development, so I include both in the following lists of developmental milestones.

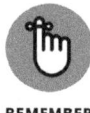

REMEMBER

As you examine any developmental checklist, keep in mind that developmental "rules" don't apply to all kids, and development isn't predestined. The path each child takes is predicable yet unique. Pediatricians are experts in watching kids grow at their own rate and pace, and within their own ability. The goal is to anticipate and prepare for the next phase, while appreciating the phase your child is in. If you're ever concerned about your child's developmental progress, your pediatrician should be your first call.

Toddlers (2–4 years)

The task of toddlerhood is to develop basic social and emotional skills. During these years, toddlers begin to show a wider range of emotional expression, such as joy, anger, frustration, and empathy. However, they struggle to express these emotions verbally. This can lead to behaviors like temper tantrums as they learn to assert their independence within necessary safety boundaries. Kids in this age range typically achieve the following social-emotional milestones in the approximate order, over time:

» Engages in symbolic pretend play, substituting objects for other things

» Has bedtime fears and nightmares

» Initiates interactions with a few peers

» Understands simple rules

» Is able to talk about emotions and situations that elicit them

» Identifies rules for problem-solving, trying solutions before getting frustrated

» Generalizes rules from one situation to another, sometimes incorrectly

» Offers comfort to another person who is hurting

» Expresses guilt for misbehaving

» Understands moral themes (right and wrong) in stories

» Plays with 3–4 peers with cooperation and sharing skills, more complex play and elaborate pretend play evolve with little distinction between fantasy and reality

Early childhood (5–7 years)

During early childhood, kids begin to develop more social and emotional skills. They start to understand and manage their emotions better, but still need support. Cooperation, sharing, and conflict resolution among friendships become more refined. Social dynamics like peer approval and fitting in become important. Self-esteem begins to form based on interactions with others.

The following are a few of the social-emotional milestones gained over these years:

>> Shows increasing emotional regulation over anger and aggression

>> Resolves conflicts with discussion and negotiation

>> Takes turns in conversation, responds appropriately

>> Initiates separation from parents, plays away for several hours in another room

>> Follows group rules, understands games with rules

>> Develops a sense of conscience, insists on rules with peers

>> Displays emotions other than the one felt underneath, or "hides" emotions

>> Continues moral development

>> Develops more complex coping skills

>> Takes responsibility for household chores with deeper understanding of their role within the family

Middle childhood (8–11 years)

In middle childhood, kids develop a stronger sense of self. They become better at managing their emotions, understanding others' perspectives, and resolving conflicts independently. Friendships become more meaningful and are based on shared interests, loyalty, and trust. During this phase, children also start to experience a deeper awareness of social norms and how their behavior affects others, which contributes to a growing sense of responsibility and empathy.

Social-emotional milestones in this life phase include the following:

>> Begins to prefer peers over family

>> Continues to build resilience through supportive adult relationships

>> Navigates more complex social interactions with the support of adults, like disagreements, breakups, and new friendships

>> Creates increasingly stable friendships based on similar interests, trust, and loyalty

>> Begins to form their identity based on achievements, social feedback, and how they view their abilities

>> Takes more interest in group activities, like sports and clubs, providing opportunities for collaboration and social learning

Recognizing Challenges in Pediatric Mental Health

Kids aren't little adults, and a pediatrician's job is to work and care for this moving masterpiece. This work has inherent challenges, especially when working toward mental health goals. It's not uncommon that as the brain grows, one symptom resolves or a challenge is overcome, only to leave a new issue in its wake. Sometimes, these changes add clarity. Other times, they are unexpected and befuddling. This is growing up.

Understanding and interpreting emotions are exceptionally difficult and individualized skills. For example, something that makes one child fearful may have no effect on another. Patience, with consistent emotional guidance, is necessary.

Emotional expression takes decades to develop. Learning to express emotion is more than just knowing the words or labeling with colors. Without life experience and higher-level brain parts, the interpretation and expression of emotion is inconsistent and incomplete. Understanding and supporting your child requires meeting them at their developmental stage and not overlaying adult-level context onto your kids' words and experiences.

Outlandish or extreme behaviors that may embarrass adults are developmentally normal for young kids. Because children are naturally self-centered, their actions can sometimes seem offensive or rude — but they don't reflect a broken moral compass or a lack of family values. It isn't until after puberty that kids develop the ability to reflect on their experiences, gain perspective, and compare their lives to others.

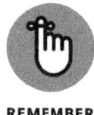

REMEMBER

You are not alone. Healthcare providers are here to support and help all families, with the shared goal of raising emotionally mature adults. Being open and honest with your pediatrician about your concerns regarding your child's social-emotional growth will enhance your visits and help you build trusted support.

Chapter **3**

Knowing Your Family Isn't Alone

As you try to understand childhood anxiety and how it may be affecting your family, rest assured that you're not alone. Millions of kids with anxiety live in families just like yours. The good news is that identifying and supporting anxious kids will lessen the negative effects of its symptoms, and it's never too late to help.

In this chapter, you recognize the vast number of children and their families who are living with anxiety. I share a few of the common reasons that anxiety is prevalent in childhood, including both biological and environmental factors, and why it may be on the rise. Finally, you realize how the support of your family is intertwined with your child's experience with anxiety.

Anxious Kids Are Everywhere

Anxiety disorders are among the most commonly diagnosed mental health conditions in children and adolescents around the world. One recent meta-analysis of 41 studies across 27 countries suggests the worldwide prevalence of anxiety disorders in 6- to 18-year-olds is 6.5 percent. In the United States, recent data from the Centers for Disease Control and Prevention (CDC) indicate 8.6 percent of children ages 6 to 11 have a diagnosed anxiety disorder.

The number of kids with anxiety is staggering. At current rates, if you were to fill a school bus, five of the riders would have an anxiety diagnosis. In a standard elementary school of 600 kids, 50 are struggling with symptoms of anxiety. A birthday party of 12 kids? At least one of the guests is suffering from overwhelming worry. And if you picked up this book, the odds are that *your kid* is that one.

Here's the point. If you're living with a young person who has irrational or uncontrollable worries and fears, you aren't alone. As isolating, confusing, or stressful this season of your parenting may feel, millions of parents around the world are sharing this experience with you. Even more importantly, with your love, support, and guidance, there are ways your child can feel better.

REMEMBER

Anxiety is universal. It happens in people from all socioeconomic classes, ethnicities, and education levels. Experiencing this common and important feeling shouldn't evoke any shame or embarrassment in yourself or your kids.

Exploring the Rise in Child Anxiety

As normal as the experience of anxiety is, the dramatic rise in young children with anxiety disorders is a global concern. In 2021, the U.S. Surgeon General issued an advisory highlighting the rapidly rising rates of anxiety and other mental health issues in young people. In turn, researchers have been investigating the reasons for this surge. The following sections discuss a few of the current findings.

Advancing science

Decades ago, anxiety in children was dismissed as shyness, nervousness, or "just a phase." Today, childhood anxiety disorders are recognized as diagnosable medical conditions that require intervention. This evolution has taken place through advancing research in child psychology and brain development, including studies demonstrating differences in brain activity among anxious children. This work validates anxiety as a neurobiological condition rather than just a behavior.

As a result of neuroscience research, evidence-supported recommendations have increased the ability of schools, pediatricians, and parents to screen for anxiety and recognize warning signs. This awareness is allowing more children to be diagnosed and supported. In addition, this research has validated the use of various therapies and treatments to bring childhood anxiety into remission, leading to a more natural increase in families seeking the diagnosis to begin successful treatment.

Normalizing mental health

In the past, openly discussing childhood anxiety was rare. Now, mental health is a mainstream conversation. Parents are disclosing mental health challenges, seeking treatment, and discussing the diagnosis with their families. Many schools now have mental health counselors, and pediatricians regularly discuss anxiety, making early intervention the norm. With this open awareness comes less stigma, better support, positive coping strategies, and treatment options for kids who are struggling.

TIP

Talking about mental health helps kids recognize and manage it. When you approach anxiety with reassurance and problem-solving, kids become less anxious, not more. Ask your child directly about their feelings. These conversations reduce shame, build confidence, and foster resilience — exactly what every child needs.

Increasing screen time

Screens aren't inherently bad, but excessive use is linked to rising anxiety in young children. Too much screen time reduces healthy peer interactions, increases exposure to bullying and negative news, and fosters social isolation. Social media can set unrealistic expectations and lead to unhealthy comparisons. Screens also disrupt emotional regulation pathways in the brain, making anxiety harder to manage.

Screen time interferes with the things in life that buffer anxiety's negative effects. Specifically, screens interfere with protective sleep, displace time meant for unstructured play, crowd out coping skill practice, and disrupt peer and family connection. Of course, these screen time effects are not just on the kids, but you, too!

TIP

Managing screen time wisely to mitigate its risks is part of modern parenting life. Find successful screen time strategies in Chapter 13.

Acknowledging the pandemic effect

The sudden isolation, disrupted routines, and prolonged stress during the COVID-19 pandemic, which began in 2020, heightened anxiety in children around the world. School closures and restricted activities affected their ability to learn and connect with peers, while dramatically increasing time in front of screens. Kids felt the strain of family financial struggles, job loss, and uncertainty; millions of children faced death and tragedy as loved ones got sick and died. As a result, today's kids are more aware of global crises than previous generations. As history unfolds, researchers will continue to uncover the long-term effects of the virus and our response to it.

Amplifying background stressors

It's easy to forget that it's hard to be a kid. Today's kids are being raised in a very demanding, high-achieving environment. Early academic pressure and frequent standardized testing contribute to anxiety. Not uncommonly, after-school activities are a source of chronic stress, while limiting kids' ability to have unstructured play and downtime. Meanwhile, running around from activity to activity often disrupts formative and protective routines, like family meals and consistent bedtimes.

Increasing parental stress

Today's parents face unprecedented levels of stress and anxiety fueled by economic pressures, political tension, and information overload. Modern parents are balancing demanding careers with household and parenting responsibilities, often with little meaningful support. Additionally, the social media–driven competitive parenting culture emphasizes achievement and milestones, leading to overscheduling, micromanaging, and excessive concern over normal childhood struggles.

Rising parental anxiety, burnout, and mental exhaustion are also significantly shaping the emotional well-being of children. When parents are overwhelmed, hypervigilant, or catastrophizing, children internalize that the world is unsafe. In addition, when parents are stressed, their emotional availability is disrupted, making it harder for parents to model regulated behavior for kids. Addressing parental well-being can help break the cycle, allowing kids to develop confidence and resilience instead of inheriting anxiety.

Predicting Anxiety

Although it feels overwhelming, rising childhood anxiety isn't a doomsday message. Kids are more capable, adaptive, and resilient than most adults give them credit for. But taking a deeper look into the multilayered reasons why kids are struggling helps break down the problem into smaller pieces, and expose ways that you can help.

Anxiety results from a complex blend of influences, each no more or less important than the others. These influences appear to be additive with genetic, environmental, and individual risk factors combining in unique ways to increase the likelihood of diagnosis, severity, and lifelong recurrence. With this context in mind, the following sections explore key factors that predict anxiety in kids.

Developing brains and anxiety symptoms

A child's experience with social-emotional regulation changes as they grow. Chapter 2 emphasizes the expected progression of a young child's social-emotional development, which reflects the maturation of specific brain parts. As the brain grows, there are stages where normal brain development creates natural imbalances in emotional and cognitive development, creating windows where anxiety symptoms are most likely to present.

Anxiety evolves as children grow. In early childhood, separation anxiety and phobias are most common. By middle childhood, generalized and social anxiety emerge, and phobias persist. Panic disorder typically appears in adolescence. Chapter 4 covers these diagnoses in detail. This natural progression of anxiety's presentation makes identification and treatment more appropriately targeted to a child's developmental phase.

Sharing genetics and epigenetics

Genetics play a role in the development of anxiety. Just like traits such as eye color or height, the tendency toward anxious thinking and sensitivity to stress can run in families. Studies with twin siblings have shown that if one parent has anxiety, the risk of a child developing anxiety is higher. The contribution of a child's genetic risk to develop an anxiety disorder is estimated to be 30–50 percent.

Emerging research in *epigenetics* is helping to explain how a child's genes are expressed over time. Epigenetics is the study of how your environment and experiences can turn genes on or off without changing the actual DNA sequence, like a light switch controlling how brightly a bulb shines. In the context of anxiety disorders, epigenetic research shows that chronic stress and tension can activate or suppress certain genes related to emotional regulation, shaping a child's brain to process fear, threats, and safety.

For example, a child who lives in a consistently high-stress or unpredictable environment may develop heightened sensitivity to stress because the genes responsible for calming the nervous system aren't "turned on" effectively. Research is finding that stress, trauma, or even a parent's mental health can change how genes work, making a child more or less likely to develop anxiety.

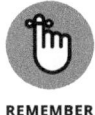

REMEMBER

What's encouraging about this science is that positive experiences, like emotional support, effective therapy, and healthy coping skills, can switch genes in a way that helps kids manage stress and build resilience. This means that even if a child has a genetic tendency toward anxiety, positive daily experiences shape how their genes behave, offering hope for healthy growth.

Appreciating child temperament

Genetics also contribute to a child's *temperament,* or an attribute that defines the child's approach to the world. Temperament is the "style" or "personality" a child is born with. It influences a child's behavior, interaction with others, and perception of the world. Temperament can't be changed and is often recognizable as early as infancy.

Researchers have categorized temperament into three broad groups: easy or flexible, active or feisty, and slow-to-warm or cautious. Of course, individual children aren't going to cleanly fit into one of the three categories. However, in most people, one temperament is most dominant.

Children with a cautious temperament, called *behavioral inhibition (BI),* are seven times more likely to develop an anxiety disorder. Kids with BI are born with an overactive fear system that leads to inflexibility. As toddlers, they show strong separation anxiety, intense meltdowns, and heightened vigilance in new situations. In middle childhood, they are shy and "slow to warm up." As they grow, they become overly focused on their performance and constantly evaluate themselves in social situations.

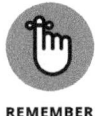

REMEMBER

No matter which temperament your child may have, environmental factors can influence how their temperament presents. The most fearful toddlers can learn to tolerate stress over time, and a laid-back kindergartener can become overly rigid, based on the world around them. What every kid needs, regardless of temperament, is support and guidance from caring adults.

Looking at parenting style

Kids aren't raised in a vacuum; they reflect the support provided by their caregivers at home. Young children are constantly looking to the adults around them for clues on how to interpret and respond to everyday challenges. In turn, your parenting style takes a powerful role in shaping your child's emotional world.

Research has repetitively found that overcontrolling parental behaviors can be a predictor of anxiety in a child. Additionally, having overly critical parents is connected with constant fear in adolescence. Conversely, the relationship between BI and the development of anxiety behaviors can be lessened by using supporting and positive parenting practices. Chapter 12 details the strengths of each parenting style and how modification to parenting styles can help foster strong parent-child relationships.

Accepting Your Child's Anxiety

If you think your child is suffering from anxiety, or your child has been recently diagnosed, it's normal to have a kaleidoscope of emotions. After I've diagnosed anxiety in a young child, parents will commonly express sadness, blame, or defeat. Sometimes, tears uncontrollably fall. All these feelings — and more — are valid. When your child is experiencing something painful or uncomfortable, it's normal to hold uncertainty and fear. However, it should be clear that your child's anxiety isn't something you could have prevented or something you can control. Your child needs your support and love as they learn to understand this part of themselves.

REMEMBER

As you read this book, you discover that anxiety is a biologically driven diagnosis that is common, diagnosable, and treatable — regardless of the trigger or primary cause. The more quickly you understand and accept your child's anxiety as a medical diagnosis, rather than a character trait or "problem," the sooner you're able to develop a comprehensive plan for treatment and remission.

Identifying anxiety early matters

Untreated anxiety disorders that begin early in life can become chronic and are associated with a high probability of recurrence. This unremitting pattern can lead to a lifetime struggle with mental health. Chapter 4 details how anxiety impacts all areas of a child's life from academics and sports to family and peer relationships. The longer a young child's life is interrupted by anxiety symptoms, the more their future may be impacted.

When anxiety is identified early, kids can learn healthy ways to cope before anxious patterns become more deeply rooted. Things like effective parenting strategies, evidence-based therapy, and school collaboration can reduce distress and help your child feel more confident and capable as they grow. You aren't overreacting by paying attention to early signs of anxiety; you're giving your child the tools they need to flourish.

REMEMBER

The expression of anxiety changes over time, making some phases more easily identifiable than others. Support at any age is helpful to long-term anxiety experience.

Reframing your role

You can't take anxiety away from your child. It's part of their life experience, brain pathways, and developmental growth. Your job is to offer understanding, support, and love. Reading this book is your first step. Hopefully, these pages will inspire you to reach out to the professional support your child may need, while optimizing your support at home.

REMEMBER

Ignoring your child's struggles would mean missing the chance to help — but you're not doing that. You're choosing to understand, support, and guide them toward healing. You're proving to yourself and your child that you see their struggles and are committed to finding healthy solutions. You're showing them love through your actions.

IN THIS CHAPTER

» **Revealing anxiety's complexity**

» **Discovering the three domains of anxiety disorder**

» **Differentiating adult from childhood anxiety**

» **Checking out child anxiety disorder types**

» **Understanding why identification matters**

Chapter **4**

Seeing What Anxiety Looks Like in Kids

A nxiety is the most common childhood mental health condition, affecting about 7 percent worldwide. In the United States, an estimated 1 in 12 children experience anxiety, which aligns with my daily work as a pediatrician. While taking care of kids of all ages, I've seen the many ways anxiety can appear throughout childhood and how kids ultimately thrive.

In this chapter, you discover why child anxiety is difficult for parents to identify and pediatricians to diagnose. I introduce the three domains of anxiety and the various types of anxiety disorders commonly seen in children. Finally, you take to heart the importance of identifying childhood anxiety by appreciating its lifelong consequences if untreated.

Recognizing That Anxiety Is the Greatest Mimicker

In my pediatric practice, kids don't walk into my office and say, "Hey, Doc. I think I'm anxious." Instead, kids with anxiety say the following:

>> "My tummy hurts in the morning."

>> "It's hard to get to sleep at night."

>> "I'm getting headaches at school."

>> "My eyes are doing weird things."

>> "My heart hurts during math class."

In the following sections, I share two patient stories that include these clues. Both children show signs of anxiety, but their diagnoses emerge in different ways. These stories show how uniquely anxiety appears in children and how spotting it often takes careful attention and detective work.

Introducing two different case studies

Grace and Reed are two patients who are visiting my office on a busy Friday afternoon. First, 6-year-old Grace arrives with her parents. This is her story:

> Grace has been complaining of stomachaches almost daily for the past two months. She describes her pain as squeezing around her belly button that sometimes makes her skip dinner or sit out during recess at school. The pain doesn't seem to wake her at night, and she denies constipation. Her mother has tried giving her over-the-counter antacids and changing her diet, but nothing has helped. Her parents are worried that something is wrong because celiac disease runs in the family.

> During the visit, Grace was clingy with her parents but allowed me to do a physical exam, which was unremarkable. We agreed that screening her for celiac disease was a good first step. Meanwhile, I asked the family to keep a more detailed record of when she complained of pain.

At her follow-up visit, her lab work was reassuringly normal. But by keeping a closer record of her tummy complaints, a pattern developed. Grace most consistently complained of her pain on Sunday night and Monday morning. In addition, her teacher had reached out and said she's visiting the nurse's office nearly every day at around 2 p.m. — the same time as her most difficult subject. At this point, the diagnosis became clearer.

Shortly after, Reed, an athletic 10-year-old, arrives with his mom. His mom leads the following conversation:

"Reed is very smart and great at basketball. Since the beginning of school, however, we've had more problems. The teachers report that he's not paying attention and spacing out during class. His grades are down, and he is not showing any motivation to make any changes. Now that basketball season has started, the coach says that he's not playing as aggressively and taking too many water breaks. All of this is very different than last year, and I know he's not living up to his potential."

Reed was quiet during most of the visit, but did mention that he's been having more headaches recently. Mom attributed this to his refusal to drink from his water bottle in class; it always comes home full. Reed said that his head gets better when he drinks water during practice; that's why he's taking more breaks.

During the visit screening tools were offered to Reed, his mom, and his teachers. The results indicated inattention. At this point, his mom agreed to start seeing a therapist and consider medical management for his ADHD. I coached Reed on how much water to drink and other headache-relieving options.

Two months later, he was back in my office. Everything was worse. His therapist determined there was more going on than Reed had initially expressed.

Hunting for clues

Grace and Reed are both struggling with anxiety. However, as you can imagine from the wildly different symptoms, Grace and Reed took very different paths to reach their diagnosis.

Grace was first evaluated for abdominal pain before addressing her anxiety. Reed was initially diagnosed with attention-deficit/hyperactivity disorder (ADHD), but his anxiety surfaced only after his symptoms worsened with medication. For both, weeks were spent exploring other potential causes before identifying anxiety as the primary issue. These detours were not mistakes but part of a thorough evaluation process tailored to each child's needs.

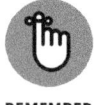
REMEMBER

Diagnosing childhood anxiety is often a winding road. Anxiety symptoms mimic many other medical and psychological issues, which makes getting the diagnosis a time-consuming process. Although your pediatrician shares the goal of helping your child feel better quickly, evaluating the symptoms of anxiety requires persistence, patience, and collaboration.

REMEMBER

Being an advocate for your child requires mental flexibility to consider all options. Your pediatrician isn't going to jump to the diagnosis of anxiety, and you shouldn't either.

Looking for a chameleon

REMEMBER

At its core, anxiety is an uncontrollable set of symptoms or behaviors triggered by a task or experience that feels threatening. However, young kids often can't make the connection between their brain and behavior or describe how they feel. As a result, most kids *show* anxiety in a variety of ways, including

>> Avoidance of certain academic or social situations

>> Physical complaints

>> Changes in sleep

>> Worrying excessively

>> Worsening school performance

>> Explosive or defiant behavior

>> Changes in eating habits

>> Suicidal thoughts or behaviors, even in the absence of depression

To complicate matters, children can consciously or unconsciously suppress the outward expression of anxiety. A child struggling with anxiety may engage in *avoidance behaviors,* or actions to escape things that cause unwanted stress or discomfort, often without a parent's awareness. This allows the child to blend in, making the symptoms less obvious.

Monitoring for misdirection

In child psychiatry, behavioral and emotional problems are grouped into two large categories, *internalizing* and *externalizing.* Anxiety is an internalizing behavior, focusing on the self. Other examples include depression, social withdrawal, and low self-esteem. In contrast, externalizing behaviors, like aggression, impulsiveness, defiance, and rule violation, are directed toward other people and the social environment.

Internalizing behaviors are harder to notice. Kids with these behaviors are often shy, withdrawn, and quiet, and they keep to themselves. Because they aren't as disruptive, these behaviors are much less noticeable than externalizing behaviors. Even the best parents can miss internalizing behaviors; it's impossible to read someone else's mind.

The challenge in children is that anxiety can resemble an externalizing disorder. When a child feels threatened, their stress response can be explosive. Fear activates the brain's fight-or-flight response, causing a stressed-out kid to cry, yell, or misbehave in school, which may make anxiety look like something else. Additionally, anxiety often co-exists with other behavioral disorders, like ADHD and obsessive-compulsive disorder (OCD), making it difficult to identify the root cause of a child's distress.

REMEMBER

Kids are constantly changing, and what you observe can vary from day to day and over time. Don't be discouraged if you feel like you've "missed" your child's anxiety. Getting the diagnosis leads to effective treatment, regardless of your child's age or experience.

REMEMBER

Fully understanding the complexity of a child's brain and body requires careful observation, open-mindedness, and collaboration with your child's trusted healthcare team. Getting the diagnosis often involves unexpected shifts, but the predictable and persistent symptoms of childhood anxiety will eventually become clear. The journey to the diagnosis is part of the process.

Understanding Anxiety's Three Parts

Child anxiety can be understood by examining its emotional, behavioral, and physical aspects. Diagnosing anxiety typically involves elements of all three, though not all may appear in every child. The following sections explore each aspect and how they contribute to anxiety.

Emotional

An *emotion* is a complex psychological state that is a response to something happening to you. For our purposes in this book, emotions are considered *innate* or hardwired into our brain and present from birth. The basic emotions — happiness, sadness, surprise, anger, fear, and disgust — are used as building blocks for more complex emotions like love, compassion, shame, and jealousy.

Emotions are universal to all humans across the world and essential for communication and survival. Primary emotions are automatic, instinctual, and intense responses to stimuli. As we grow, culture and individual experiences can influence our emotions. In this way, emotions are adaptive, helping us respond to our environment and guiding decision-making.

Emotions are intricately related to *feelings,* which are the conscious experience and interpretation of an emotion. Feelings are powerful and persuasive, especially in young kids. However, how we interpret emotions isn't always correct. Our life experiences, circumstances, and the people around us shape our interpretation. These influences can distort facts, overgeneralize, catastrophize, or project personal thoughts, making our feelings real and valid but also inaccurate and misleading.

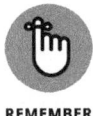

Emotions are raw data, and *feelings* are how we interpret and make sense of the data.

The emotional component of anxiety shows up as excessive worry or fear about situations that seem commonplace to others, like going to school, making friends, or trying something new. Over time, this worry is increasingly difficult to control. Often, kids struggle to identify or explain what they are worried about. Because explaining emotions with words is difficult — even for adults — kids express emotion through behaviors.

Anxiety is a *feeling* rooted in the primary *emotion* of fear.

Behavioral

Behavior is an outward sign of emotion. Voluntary behaviors include facial expressions, body language, or actions; involuntary behaviors, like sweating or blinking, occur without conscious thought. Observing behavioral changes is easy, but interpreting them correctly requires keen, contextual observations over time.

Anxiety affects how kids behave. Anxious behaviors interfere with a child's ability to best function at school, home, or with friends. Key anxiety behaviors include avoiding feared activities and seeking excessive reassurance. Other behaviors common to child anxiety include the following:

>> Crying

>> Tantrums

>> Clinging to a caregiver

>> Reluctance to engage with certain people

>> Running away or freezing

>> Aggression toward others

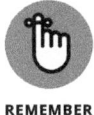

Crying, irritability, or tantrums are often quickly interpreted by parents as defiance or disobedience. In kids with anxiety, however, these behaviors are a natural stress response. Understanding the context of your child's outbursts is crucial for making this distinction.

Physical

Anxiety doesn't stay in the brain; it affects the body. The brain regions and neurotransmitters involved in anxiety have wide-ranging functions in the human body, many of which are unrelated to psychological disorders. It's these *somatic,* or "body," symptoms of anxiety that bring kids to my office. Somatic symptoms are often complex, occurring during both times of stress and perceived calm. Ultimately, it's the uncomfortable physical symptoms that young anxious kids complain about and want to go away.

REMEMBER

Physical discomfort creates anxiety, and anxiety creates physical discomfort. Addressing your child's physical symptoms directly is a necessary part of a complete anxiety management plan. Be sure to ask your doctor what you can do to improve your child's physical symptoms.

In Chapter 5, I discuss how the physical symptoms of anxiety manifest from the stress response's activation of the nervous system. Common physical signs of child anxiety include

>> Sweating

>> Heart racing

>> Chest tightness

>> Abdominal pain or nausea

>> Feeling lightheaded or faint

>> Chills or body tremors

>> Muscle tightness

The physical symptoms of many diseases overlap with the symptoms of anxiety. It's important to include a physical evaluation when considering mental health conditions to rule out primary medical problems. You can find out more about medical problems that mimic anxiety and how to support your child during a medical exam in Chapters 6 and 7.

Noticing How Child Anxiety Differs from Adult Anxiety

Anxiety is a protective mechanism created by the brain through a blend of neurochemistry, physiology, and environment. In both adults and children, these elements influence how anxiety is expressed. However, as I mention in Chapter 2, kids aren't little adults. Their immature neurophysiology, innate temperament, and environment make the development and expression of anxiety in children exceptionally unique.

Physiology

Anxiety symptoms result from an imbalance between the thinking and emotional areas of a child's brain. The *prefrontal cortex* (PFC), part of the thinking brain, helps plan, predict, make decisions, and manage social behaviors. A fully developed PFC interprets emotional input and slows down the fast-acting *limbic system*, or emotional brain, which includes the *amygdala*. The amygdala controls defensive behavior, fear expression, and fear-related memories. The strength of the connection between the PFC and the amygdala plays a key role in the type and severity of anxiety. (For more on brain structure and neurotransmitters, see Chapter 2.)

In kids, the emotional brain develops before the thinking brain. Because the PFC doesn't mature until adulthood, the emotional amygdala is effectively unchecked, resulting in explosive emotional responses and reactions. The largest naturally occurring functional imbalance between PFC and amygdala happens during adolescence. This may be a hallmark clue to the development of anxiety as a teen.

REMEMBER

Anxiety is one of the most common childhood mental health disorders. Understanding more about the physiology and biology of the condition helps us have greater compassion for our kids who may be struggling.

Neurotransmitters, like serotonin and dopamine, are chemical messengers that help the thinking and emotional brain communicate. Changes in neurotransmitter activity can increase or decrease anxiety symptoms and behaviors. A young child's brain is more sensitive to certain neurotransmitters than an adult's brain. Additionally, some systems that regulate neurotransmitter processing aren't fully developed, leading to chemical differences. These factors make the experience and expression of anxiety unique in young children.

TECHNICAL
STUFF

In young children, anxiety most often appears before depressive symptoms. Depression involves more complex thought patterns that require higher brain development. Young kids typically lack the brain development needed for self-reflection and abstract reasoning associated with depression.

Temperament

A child's temperament, their natural way of thinking, feeling, and behaving, affects how anxiety is expressed. Temperament acts as a built-in personality blueprint that makes each child unique. Some kids are naturally calm and easygoing, and others are more energetic, cautious, or sensitive. Although temperament is something a child is born with, it can change as they grow and learn from experiences.

Temperament traits can be identified as early as infancy. Children who are naturally apprehensive, hesitant, or easily upset by new experiences are considered *behaviorally inhibited* (BI). This BI temperament is linked to physiological traits, like higher stress hormone levels, that remain stable throughout childhood. As they grow, behaviorally inhibited children are more likely to develop anxiety. (Find out more about childhood temperament in Chapter 3.)

Temperament persists in adulthood and continues to influence anxiety development and stress management. However, unlike children, adults have a more developed cognitive brain, enabling adults to suppress unwanted behaviors and apply effective coping skills. Adults also have self-awareness and social influences to help modify their actions, abilities that children do not yet possess.

Environment

Environmental factors dramatically influence the expression of anxiety. Kids don't choose the family they are born into, the zip code in which they live, or where they go to school. A child's growth and development is a direct reflection of life circumstances largely outside of their control.

Most kids grow up in a loving, nurturing environment surrounded by family, friends, teachers, and coaches. However, some children face environments where adults lack the emotional, physical, or financial capacity to care for them. Others experience bullying, strict academic pressures, or natural disasters. Additionally, every child is vulnerable to unexpected accidents, illnesses, injuries, or trauma. During childhood's formative years, stressful situations have the power to strengthen the mental pathways responsible for fear and anxiety.

Difficulty regulating fear and learning fear responses are central features of anxiety. Anxiety thought patterns begin developing early in childhood. Kids interpret context and safety cues uniquely, influenced by their surroundings. They learn fear-based responses through direct negative experiences, false alarms, or by observing others' fear reactions. Over time, unlearning or ignoring these threat associations becomes very challenging.

REMEMBER

You are your child's external brain. Your reactions and guidance help your child interpret and navigate their surroundings.

Time span

As the brain develops, the presentation of anxiety changes. For example, a teenager with generalized anxiety disorder may have experienced severe separation anxiety as a young child.

Certain phases of brain growth are also more sensitive to the biological and neurotransmitter imbalances that contribute to anxiety symptoms. To an observant parent, this means anxiety in a child can appear to move into and out of various forms over the years.

Interestingly, gene expression changes throughout childhood as the brain moves through different developmental stages. During various phases, certain genes that influence anxiety become more or less active. This natural shift is another way to explain why anxiety can look different as kids grow, with genetics playing a stronger role in early and middle childhood and lessening over time.

Distinguishing Types of Child Anxiety Disorders

Kids with anxiety disorders have maladaptive, fear-dominated thinking patterns that lead to emotional distress and avoidance behaviors. Consistent with all types of anxiety is fear that is out of proportion with the situation, person, object, event, or threat. The context and situation where excessive worry presents helps to distinguish between the anxiety disorders.

Each type of anxiety disorder is characterized by unique features and neurobiology. Interestingly, due to brain growth and the different developmental stages it undergoes, anxiety types tend to present themselves in a predictable order. The following sections introduce each type of disorder in the order in which they are commonly seen in young children, from youngest to oldest.

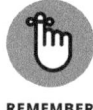

REMEMBER

Anxiety disorders in childhood commonly co-exist with other anxiety disorders. Research suggests that up to 60 percent of kids with anxiety have a blend of separation anxiety disorder, generalized anxiety disorder, and social anxiety disorder, called the "triad." In addition, anxiety disorders frequently co-occur with other psychiatric disorders of childhood, including ADHD, oppositional defiant disorder, autism spectrum disorder, language disorders, learning disabilities, and teenage depression.

Note: The names and characteristics of specific anxiety disorders have evolved over time. Psychiatry, like all medical sciences, continually refines itself based on new research and therapeutic advancements. Although the names of anxiety disorders have subtly changed over the decades, their main characteristics have remained the same.

Specific phobias

Specific phobias are one of the first anxiety disorders to appear in kids, at an average age of 6 years. A phobia is a fear related to a common situation or focus that is out of proportion to the actual danger posed by the object or situation. To be diagnosed with a phobia, the fear must be persistent and last for more than six months.

Phobias are related to fear-based anxiety disorders including separation and social anxiety, and often present with another type of anxiety disorder. In contrast to adults with specific phobias, children with phobias don't need to recognize their fear as unreasonable. Common phobias in childhood are fear of animals, environmental events, injuries, illness, blood, and injections.

TIP

One of the most common phobias I see in my office is the fear of needles. Find out how to help with needle phobia in Chapter 18.

As an example, it's normal for children to fear thunderstorms. These kids are briefly concerned and easily calmed by those around them. However, a child with a phobia of bad weather, or *astraphobia,* will get visibly anxious if the weather report mentions rain or thunder, constantly check weather apps, ask their teachers repetitive questions about the possibility of rain, and refuse to play outside at recess when dark clouds are in the sky. For more examples of normal fears versus phobias see Chapter 5.

Separation anxiety disorder

As the name implies, separation anxiety disorder (SAD) is characterized by extreme stress when a child is separated from their caregivers. This distress is recurrent, anticipatory, persistent, and lasts for at least four weeks. SAD typically appears around age 7. Females are more at risk of SAD than males, and having SAD as a child strongly increases the risk of having generalized anxiety disorder later in life.

Children with SAD often report that something bad is going to happen if they are separated from their parents, including during the night. These kids often have difficulty getting to sleep on their own, sleep with their parents, or require a parent to lie down with them while they fall asleep. Older children avoid camps and sleepovers, complaining of excessive homesickness. In addition, kids with SAD have physical symptoms during separation, most commonly stomachaches.

TIP

One way to determine if your child's behavior is normal is simply by their age. For example, separation anxiety in toddlers is a normal developmental phase. Separation anxiety *disorder* is in older kids, when they are "too old" to still be in that developmental phase. Normal developmental phases are reviewed in Chapters 2 and 5.

Selective mutism

Selective mutism (SM) is generally thought to be a rare condition, affecting about 1 percent of school-aged children. Children with SM talk readily at home and with certain close friends, but they refuse to speak at school or other settings where there is an expectation for speaking. This often presents in the years of early education.

Kids with SM don't initiate conversations or respond to people when spoken to in specific situations, with minimal associated physical symptoms. At home, they are chatterboxes with a great depth of language. To be diagnosed, the behavior has to be observed for at least four weeks (not the first four weeks of school) and interfere with a child's social or educational progress.

SM is closely linked to social anxiety disorder (see the section "Social anxiety disorder" later in this chapter), but it can also involve challenges in language learning or emerging characteristics of autism spectrum disorder. Like social anxiety disorder, studies suggest that children with SM often have a behavioral inhibition temperament from a young age. Additionally, many children with SM experience impairments in social-emotional skills or language development. These deficits improve over time with proper support and treatment.

Generalized anxiety disorder

The diagnosis of generalized anxiety disorder (GAD) includes excessive worry about various things, along with one or more of the following symptoms: restlessness, fatigue, difficulty concentrating, irritability, muscle tension, and sleep changes. These symptoms occur on most days of the week for at least six months. GAD is more common in females than in males, affecting about 3 percent of adolescents. It typically begins in school-aged children, with the average age of onset being around 9 years.

A child with GAD experiences a range of worries that are difficult to control. They struggle to tolerate uncertainty, leading to a broad range of symptoms across different settings in their life. Often, they become preoccupied with school performance, believing they must perform perfectly and focusing on mistakes rather than successes. Other children may worry about personal and family safety, often triggered by world events. GAD in childhood is strongly linked to depression in the teen and adult years.

TIP

School refusal is not a diagnosis but rather a symptom of a variety of anxiety disorders. It's typically seen in two distinct age groups, around 5–6 years and 10–11 years. See Chapter 14 for more about school refusal.

Social anxiety disorder

Kids with social anxiety disorder (SoAD) experience intense anxiety in social situations, making it difficult for them to connect with others. They worry about embarrassing themselves, fearing that others will have negative thoughts about them if they say or do the wrong thing. Their worry focuses more on what others think of them than on their own perceptions of their performance. SoAD is strongly linked to a behavioral inhibition temperament.

A child with SoAD avoids raising their hand in class and refuses to participate in group projects. They attend extracurricular events but cling to their parents and refuse to initiate conversations with peers. These kids don't like to order in restaurants or text friends on the phone, and their eye contact is often inconsistent or limited.

In kids with SoAD, social situations are avoided to eliminate the feeling of distress. Over the years, children with untreated SoAD may have reduced social skills or language skills due to lack of developmentally appropriate experiences. SoAD is associated with developing other anxiety symptoms throughout adolescence, including adolescent school refusal. To be diagnosed, symptoms must last for at least six months with significant impairment in daily functioning.

TECHNICAL
STUFF

The fear of public speaking is a form of social anxiety disorder, not a phobia. At the core, the stress of speaking comes from being judged or scrutinized in a social situation. This is different than a phobia, in which fear is directed to a specific object or situation, like spiders or heights.

TECHNICAL
STUFF

Separation and social anxiety disorders are often talked about as one type of anxiety. They share the same symptoms, consequences, neurobiology, and treatment.

Agoraphobia

Kids with agoraphobia have a pronounced fear in particular environments, such as crowded places; being in lines; small, enclosed areas; public transportation; or generally being outside of the home alone. Kids will avoid these places or situations, fearing that they will be unable to escape or cope with the physical or embarrassing symptoms.

Agoraphobia is considered separate from specific phobias. Unlike specific phobias that occur earlier in childhood, agoraphobia more broadly impacts a child's life. The average age of diagnosis is 13 years. Agoraphobia can exist with or without panic attacks and is diagnosed after six months of consistent symptoms in at least two situations.

Agoraphobia can be difficult to identify, because it can look like separation anxiety or school refusal. The difference is that a child with separation anxiety can still happily participate in soccer practice if their mom agrees to stay on the sidelines. A child with agoraphobia cannot be calmed by Mom's presence during the practice.

Panic disorder

The last anxiety disorder to emerge is panic disorder, most often seen after puberty. Kids with panic disorder describe the events by the physical symptoms they experience, such as sweating, trembling, shortness of breath, chest pain, nausea, hot flashes, or tingling. These "attacks" happen suddenly and without warning, peaking within minutes. Part of the disorder includes the constant fear that an attack may happen at any moment, which contributes to avoidance behaviors.

Panic disorder is diagnosed after one or more attacks, with at least one month of persistent worry about additional attacks. Panic disorder as a teen significantly increases the risk of GAD and depressive disorders as an adult. In addition, panic disorders are the most genetically inheritable of anxiety disorders.

Identifying Childhood Anxiety Matters

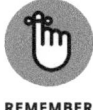

REMEMBER

Although there are different types of anxiety, diagnosis and treatment are often discussed without identifying distinctive types. Because nearly all types of anxiety disorders have similar treatment paths, delaying treatment until a specific diagnosis is reached is typically not necessary.

Untreated anxiety disorders have a profound lifelong impact on children. Anxiety shapes all areas of a child's life, including academic, social, and family functioning. The impact of anxiety on school performance is particularly significant, leading to fewer days of school attendance, less engagement, and poorer academic performance.

Among their peers and family, anxious kids are more likely to be bullied and have fewer friendships. Their anxiety symptoms often impair their ability to have successful peer relationships or cause them to be misunderstood. Anxious kids are emotionally heightened, leading to frequent arguments with family members. Plus, the stress of having an anxious child at home can strain the child-parent relationship or cause tension among caregivers.

Left untreated, anxiety has a chronic and unremitting course. Anxiety doesn't go away on its own. It may remit or lessen during periods of childhood development; however, anxiety will return as kids age into young adults and beyond. As they age, kids with anxiety are at risk for substance dependence, depression, later mood disorders, eating disorders, suicidal ideation, and early termination of their education. These all affect lifelong earning potential and contribute to adult economic disadvantages.

REMEMBER

The lifelong risks of untreated anxiety are clear. Seeking a proper diagnosis and treatment plan for your anxious child sets them up for success in young adulthood and beyond.

Identification and treatment of anxiety prevents long-term consequences. There have been exceptional strides in the last few decades in the identification and understanding of youth mental health disorders. Researchers and scientists have a much better understanding of the underlying neurobiological causes of anxiety disorders and risk factors, allowing treatments that are more personalized to the unique biology of a growing child and tailored to problem-focused solutions.

Chapter **5**

Understanding Normal Childhood Worries and Fears

Not all worry is anxiety, and not all fears are phobias. Although these emotional experiences can feel similar, there are significant differences between what's normal and what's cause for alarm. Getting insight into these feelings and behaviors helps you avoid two traps: brushing off real concerns and overreacting to a typical phase of development. In this chapter, you discover the relationship between stress and anxiety, and you identify signs of stress in kids. You classify fears and worries as normal or something else. All the while, I share ways to support your child's growing emotional awareness and development.

Appreciating the Stress Response

Experiencing worry, fear, and anxiety is a normal part of being human. Short bursts of anxiety can be productive, motivating — even helpful! Anxiety can help you hit a big deadline at work and crush your keynote speaking event. Fear protects you from an oncoming car or a charging bear. And appropriate worries about your child's health provide motivation to seek help. We need all these emotions and feelings to be a dynamic and healthy person.

Anxiety, fear, and worry all create a stress response. When we're stressed, epinephrine, norepinephrine, and cortisol stimulate the sympathetic nervous system. As I discuss in Chapter 6, nearly every cell has receptors for these powerful hormones. When triggered, they flood the bloodstream, causing a cascade of physiological changes. Though they are sometimes uncomfortable, the physical symptoms created by the stress response are essential for survival.

Different situations change how much stress hormone is released and how long the stress cascade lasts. Mild stress, like a test, triggers a small response, but a big presentation may cause a larger response. An attacking lion? That will trigger the most intense stress reaction of all — the "fight-or-flight" reaction. No matter the stressful trigger, the resulting hormone-driven stress pathway is the same. The difference between worry and anxiety, or fear and phobia, is the *duration* and *intensity* of the stress response.

REMEMBER

You can't (and shouldn't) shield your child from difficulty or change. Your love and guidance help shape their experience of life through both good and challenging times. *You* are exactly what they need!

Finding signs of stress in kids

Stress is a normal part of growing up. It's common for children to feel nervous before a test, frustrated with friends, or worried about a new situation like starting school. When children experience stress, they rarely have the words to describe what they are feeling. Instead, kids *show* stress through changes in behavior, with the severity often reflected in the intensity of the behavior shift.

REMEMBER

Some signs of stress in children include

>> Changes in eating or sleeping habits

>> Physical complaints

>> New fears

>> Increased clinginess

>> Regression of previously learned skills

>> Increased aggression

>> Negative self-talk

>> Repeated questions about the future

>> Withdrawal from peers or family

>> Changes in play behavior

>> Tantrums or crying

Figuring out whether a change in your child's behavior change is normal or a sign of anxiety requires identifying the source of stress and watching how they respond over time. It's not always easy! But the sooner you spot unhealthy, stress–driven thoughts or behaviors, the sooner you can step in with support and guidance.

Children express stress through changes in their behavior, not with words.

REMEMBER

Recognizing childhood stress

A common stressor during early childhood is becoming a big sibling. The following is Hunter's story:

> Hunter is a 4-year-old boy who has recently shown changes in behavior following the arrival of his baby sister. He has always been happy and well-adjusted, but now he has become more emotional, clingy, and irritable. Unexpectedly, he started asking for his pacifier again (which he gave up years ago) and wants to

be held all the time. He is also more prone to crying when things don't go his way.

Despite these new behaviors, Hunter is curious about his little sister. He likes to help with small tasks and put his sister to bed at night. Additionally, he still enjoys going to his familiar preschool classroom and engages with his friends during the day.

In this scenario, Hunter is experiencing normal stress in response to the arrival of his baby sister. His behaviors are common in young children who are adjusting to significant changes in the family dynamic. Consistent emotional support, special one-on-one time, and routine schedules will help Hunter feel secure during the transition.

REMEMBER

Anxiety is rooted in stress. The emotional, behavioral, and physical changes in stressed kids commonly overlap the experience of anxiety. However, unlike anxiety, stress is linked to a specific event, is relatively short-lived, and improves with reassurance, rest, or problem-solving.

Knowing It's Normal to Worry

Worry is an emotional and cognitive response to thoughts or anticipations about the future. Worry emerges when children develop the ability to think about the future and anticipate potential outcomes. For most kids, the "what-ifs" start around the age of three. The future-focused aspect of worry engages more complex brain regions and cognitive pathways, meaning toddlers and preschoolers don't worry the same way that older children do.

Worry initiates the stress response; however, it doesn't trigger anxiety's robust physical symptoms or avoidance behavior. Consider Kennedy, a 6-year-old worried about someone in her family getting sick.

Kennedy is a bright and curious 6-year-old girl. Her parents report that over the past few weeks, Kennedy has frequently asked questions like "What if Mommy or Daddy gets sick?" and

"Will I get sick too?" These worries usually come up at bedtime or when she hears someone talk about illness on TV or in conversation. Kennedy is generally well-behaved, enjoys school, and participates in activities like drawing and playing with friends, but her parents have noticed that she's become clingier and needs reassurance more frequently.

Kennedy is experiencing a common early-childhood worry. Her concerns are situational, and she's able to be comforted and return to regular activities without excessive distress. She shows no significant impairment in daily life, and her need for reassurance is typical for a child of her age.

Defining age-appropriate worries

Some of the most common worries for each age group are as follows:

>> **Preschool worries (age 3–5):** At this age, children first begin to show true worry, often about their immediate surroundings and things they don't understand. Their worries are based on things they can see and hear, rather than future concerns. With vivid imaginations, they may have real worries rooted in fantasy, often making their concerns seem simple or insignificant to adults.

>> **Early elementary school worries (age 6–8):** As school-age years begin, children develop more specific worries as they expand their awareness of the world and their role in it. They may worry about social situations, academic performance, or getting hurt. They begin to anticipate negative outcomes, such as performing poorly in a piano recital or having a doctor's appointment.

>> **Middle childhood worries (age 9–11):** Kids at this age have more complex, future-oriented worries. With a better understanding of potential outcomes and life experiences, they may worry about abstract concepts like family relationships, illness consequences, or world events. Their concerns often stem from things they hear from adults, the news, or school.

Supporting kids who worry

Worry can make children overestimate danger and underestimate their ability to cope. As a result, kids who worry need support and practice. This approach doesn't prevent worry from returning but allows your child to practice facing their worry and overcoming it. This practice requires partnership, and you're the perfect person to help! Here are some ways to support a child who worries:

>> **Validate and normalize.** Give your child your full attention, validate the worry using empathetic language, and let them know it's normal for kids to worry. For example: "It's okay to worry about things. Everyone gets worried sometimes, even grown-ups. I'm here to help."

>> **Ask questions.** Ask open-ended questions about the worry and their associated feelings to gain insight into the worry's cause and guide how to address it. Use phrasing like "Can you tell me what part of today felt the hardest or made you feel yucky?"

>> **Celebrate small wins.** For a child worried about the dark, sitting in the dark for one minute can be an accomplishment.

>> **Let kids cry.** Crying is a healthy release of stress and a way to build resiliency in the face of worry. It's okay to let kids cry.

>> **Teach with stories.** Visit the library or your local bookstore to find age-appropriate books about overcoming worry.

>> **Keep a worry doll handy.** Have your child share their worries with a doll or stuffed toy. At the end of the day, place the doll in a special place so your child knows the doll is holding their worries while they sleep.

>> **Create predictability.** Kids thrive on healthy routines and boundaries. Keeping their daily schedule as consistent as possible will encourage calm.

>> **Share your experience.** With older kids, take a minute to share a time when you had a similar worry with a positive outcome.

Differentiating worry from anxiety

Worry becomes anxiety when the stress reaction is intense, prolonged, and starts to interfere with a child's life. In addition, anxiety leads to *avoidance behaviors,* or actions that kids take to avoid stressful or uncomfortable situations, like avoiding the playground, becoming withdrawn, or daydreaming. Table 5-1 illustrates some differences between normal childhood worry and anxiety.

TABLE 5-1 **Characteristics of Normal Worry versus Anxiety**

Worry	Anxiety
Soothed by the support of a caring adult	Reassurance provides little to no effect
Consistent with a child's developmental stage	Outside of developmental age or significantly different than peers
Proportional to the situation	Overwhelming, even when the stressor is minor
Short-lived	Persists over time — weeks to months
Tied to a specific situation	No apparent cause
Doesn't interfere with daily activities or relationships	Significantly alters daily functioning
Rarely results in behavioral changes	Notable, consistent shifts in behavior
May cause brief, mild physical symptoms	Recurring, intense physical symptoms

WARNING

If your child has any persisting physical complaints, schedule a visit with their doctor to ensure there's no medical cause. Although anxiety disorders include physical symptoms, missing medically treatable conditions can have serious health consequences. Chapter 6 has more information on medical mimickers.

Looking at two real-world examples

Figuring out whether your child's worries are normal or a sign of anxiety isn't always easy. The same worry may be relatively harmless in one child but a red flag for another. You can see the differences between worry and anxiety by reading about Kay and Beckett:

> Kay is an 8-year-old girl who has recently expressed concerns about school, particularly around tests and homework. Her parents report that she occasionally says things like "I'm nervous about the math test" or "What if I don't know the answers?" Kay sometimes talks about wanting to do well and worries about making mistakes. Once she gets encouragement, she usually feels better, goes to school without resistance, and fully participates. After school, she continues to enjoy gymnastics and planning manicure parties with her classmates.

> Her classmate, Beckett, has developed a significant fear of attending school over the past few months. His parents report that every school morning is an emotional struggle. Beckett cries, begs not to go, and sometimes complains of physical symptoms like stomachaches or headaches. At school, Beckett's teacher says he avoids group activities and struggles to focus. He also frequently visits the school nurse and asks to go home. After school, he has withdrawn from soccer and stopped playing Minecraft with friends.

Kay's worries about school are developmentally appropriate and reflect normal concerns about school performance. Her worries don't interfere with her daily functioning, social interactions, or school attendance. Consistent and calm reassurance is what she needs. On the other hand, Beckett's behavior suggests an anxiety disorder. Unlike typical worries about school, Beckett's irrational and overwhelming fear interferes with his ability to attend regularly, impacts his social interactions, and causes significant distress. His avoidance signals need for professional intervention, such as therapy or behavioral support. (For more about school refusal, check out Chapter 14.)

Tackling Fears

Fear is a primary emotion. It's an intense reaction to a specific threat, triggered by the brain interpreting information from the five senses. Originating in the limbic system, fear can occur without cognitive thought. This powerful emotion can make us flee or protect ourselves from danger, even before we know what is lurking behind the corner.

Here are a few ways our bodies change physiologically during a fear-induced "fight-or-flight" stress response:

>> Increased heart rate and cardiac output

>> Redirected blood flow to the brain, arms, and legs

>> Spiked glucose levels

>> Increased oxygen consumption

>> Airway constriction

>> Decreased gut absorption

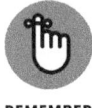

REMEMBER

We cannot control emotions, but we can control our reactions to them. All emotions provide information about our surroundings. Emotions are not inherently good or bad; they are essential for our survival.

Maturing from imaginary to reality-based fears

Young children have vivid imaginations, so early fears often revolve around "pretend" things, people within their close circle, or bad things happening to them. As kids age, the integration of their emotional and thinking brain creates more complex and reality-based fears. Table 5-2 shows common childhood fears by age.

TABLE 5-2   **Common Childhood Fears by Age**

Age (Years)	Common Fears
2–4	Fear of the dark, potty training, baths, loud noises (vacuum, thunder), shadows, animals, being away from parents
5–7	Monsters under the bed, bad guys in the closet, getting sick or hurt, nightmares, making parents mad, ghosts or supernatural things, severe weather
7–8	Fear of being left alone, death, car accidents, plane crashes, dark places
8–11	Fears about mass shootings, injuries to self or others, spiders and snakes, tests and exams, vomiting, choking, death of family members and friends

All childhood fears share the same characteristics. Childhood fears are

>> **Age-appropriate:** Fears evolve as kids grow.

>> **Short-lived:** As a child becomes more familiar with the situation or grows out of the developmental phase, the fear typically fades.

>> **Linked to specific situations:** The cause of the fear is clearly identifiable.

>> **Mildly disruptive:** Fears don't interfere with a child's ability to continue on with daily activities.

>> **Responsive to reassurance:** Over time and with support, caregiver reassurance is enough to manage and overcome the fear.

>> **Part of normal development:** Allowing children to experience and overcome fear is critical to building resiliency and understanding risk.

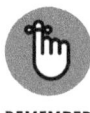

Anxiety is a complex *feeling* rooted in the primary *emotion* of fear.

REMEMBER

Helping a scared child

TIP

Kids who are fearful need you to help them lower their stress response. Over time, kids will develop the ability to acknowledge and overcome fear on their own. Here are some ways you can help:

>> **Acknowledge once, reassure once.** Over-reassurance or trying to convince them there is nothing to worry about can *confirm* a child's fear.

>> **Model calm.** Use a "ho-hum" demeanor, relaxed face, and calm tone.

>> **Use distraction.** After validating their experience, try to distract your child by talking about something else, something in the room, or something to look forward to.

>> **Allow time.** Emotions don't recondition overnight. It can take weeks to months for a child to get over a common fear.

>> **Reward small steps.** For a fearful child, any effort toward approaching the trigger is a success. Celebrate small wins to encourage self-reliance.

>> **Distinguish *realness* from *accuracy*.** The emotion of fear is real, but the danger may not be. In older kids, express this distinction by saying, "When you're scared, your brain is trying to protect you. But this feeling doesn't always mean you're in danger. Let's look at what's really going on together."

REMEMBER

Fears are a normal part of childhood, and with your support, your child can learn to navigate and overcome them.

Distinguishing fears from phobias

A fear reaction occurs within an appropriate context, diminishes when the threat is removed, and resolves on its own in about 30 minutes. When this reaction happens repeatedly, or outside what most would consider a direct threat, a phobia may be looming. Phobias in children are intense and irrational, and your child may not be able to tell you why they are scared. Phobias are long-lasting (six months or more), occur with little or no trigger, and resist reassurance. Additionally, kids with a phobia will go to great lengths to avoid the stressful trigger, creating disruptions to normal routines.

Kathryn, a healthy 10-year-old, is afraid of the dark. Do you think this is a fear or phobia?

> Kathryn's parents report that for the past few months, she becomes agitated and irritable as bedtime approaches. During tuck-in, she often begs her parents to leave the lights on. When the lights are off, she experiences shortness of breath, sweats, and feels like she's "going to die." When she finally gets to sleep, she frequently wakes during the night. In these moments, her parents can do little to reassure her, leading to irritability, fatigue, and difficulty focusing at school the next day. She is now avoiding any events that end after dark, including a slumber party with her best friend.

Kathryn's intense and persistent fear of the dark, along with regular panic attacks, avoidance behaviors, and disruption to her life, suggest a phobia rather than a typical childhood fear. Managing her phobia with professional support is the next step.

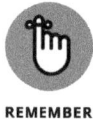

REMEMBER

Phobias during childhood are treatable. If you think your child needs help, reach out to your child's doctor for advice. Also, phobias often include panic. Find out how to support a child with panic in Chapter 16.

Chapter **6**

Watching Out for Medical Mimickers

Your child is complaining of a stomachache. Again. Your child's teacher sent an email saying they went to the school nurse three days last week. You're moving around your work schedule for the fourth time this month because they are home from school with a headache. Is this all from anxiety, or is something else going on?

In this chapter, you find out why anxiety causes a variety of physical symptoms in kids. I walk through the most common physical symptoms of anxiety, calling out associated medical conditions that mimic anxiety symptoms or issues that make anxiety worse. Additionally, I offer some practical at-home tips to help your child's symptoms improve.

REMEMBER

The following information summarizes the most common causes of various body complaints in anxious kids. This isn't meant to be an exhaustive list, and there are always exceptions to the information. The purpose of this chapter is to provide general medical advice. It doesn't establish any professional relationship between you and me. Any specific concerns, issues, or worries need to be addressed with your child's healthcare provider.

Appreciating the Brain-Body Connection

Anxiety lives in your brain and your body. The physical symptoms of anxiety, fear, and stress trigger your brain to create a flood of hormones that activate the "fight-or-flight" response throughout your entire body.

Stress hormones released during anxiety impact the body in countless ways. Stress hormones interact with the immune system, making you more prone to infections. They can also disrupt digestion, causing stomachaches, nausea, or changes in appetite. Stress-induced elevation of heart rate and blood pressure can manifest as headaches or chest pain. Over time, the repeated activation of this stress response can even change the way your brain and body handle future stressors, potentially making you more reactive to minor stress in the future.

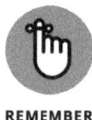

REMEMBER

Pain and discomfort triggered by anxiety is not "all in your head" — the physiologic effects of stress hormones are real, have a biological cause, and deserve attention and treatment.

In the rest of this chapter, I walk you through the most common physical symptoms of childhood anxiety. I describe the biological reasons your child's anxiety causes physical symptoms and offer ways for you to address their discomfort. Also, I share physical symptoms that are rarely associated with anxiety. My goal is to help your anxious child feel better and alert you to symptoms of significance that may require medical attention.

Responding to Tummy Troubles

One of the most common reasons kids come to my office is that their tummy hurts. Here comes Gage, a healthy 7-year-old, who arrives with his mother:

> Over the past three months, Gage has been complaining of persistent abdominal pain, which he describes as a "cramping" feeling around his belly button. The pain occurs almost daily, often during school hours, and sometimes wakes him at night. He has no vomiting, but his appetite has decreased slightly, and he occasionally feels nauseated. Gage's bowel movements are regular, but his mother notes occasional episodes of looser stools. He has not had any recent illnesses and has no significant medical history aside from seasonal allergies. His mom is worried that he has an ulcer or gut infection and wants him evaluated by a specialist.

In this scenario, Gage is experiencing *chronic abdominal pain*, or CAP. Determining the cause of CAP is difficult because the symptoms are continuous yet vague and inconsistent. But despite the difficulty, CAP is quite common and your pediatrician can help.

REMEMBER

CAP is very different from acute abdominal pain. Acute pain is the sudden, out-of-the-blue, or severe tummy pain that makes kids look and feel sick. Things like norovirus, appendicitis, urinary tract infections, and sickle cell crisis need urgent medical attention and care. If your child has acute abdominal pain, call your doctor.

Exploring the causes of CAP

The underlying causes of CAP include both organic and functional disorders:

>> *Organic* CAP has a physical or medical reason for the pain, like a problem with digestion, an infection, or inflammation. Kids with organic causes for their pain have symptoms like weight loss, poor growth, or stool changes. For anxious kids with abdominal pain, ruling out organic causes of abdominal pain may be part of the initial workup.

>> *Functional* CAP, or disorders of gut-brain interaction (DGBIs), is more common. DGBIs cause persisting pain with no identifiable structural, infectious, or biochemical abnormality. In kids with a DGBI, physical changes or stress signals in the gut are perceived as pain. These kids also have visceral *hyperalgesia,* an increased sensitivity to pain, making normal gut function feel painful.

Introducing the ENS

One of the strongest of your brain-body connections is between the brain and the gut. In fact, most kids with DGBIs have abdominal pain due to this strong linkage, and there is a physiological reason for it. Why? Let me introduce you to the ENS.

Most people don't know that the gut has its own nervous system complex, called the *enteric nervous system* (ENS). The ENS directly connects the gut to the brain's *central nervous system,* or CNS. Through this connection, the brain constantly receives signals from the gut with information about its environment. In turn, the brain is able to send responses back to various cells in the gut. Most of this two-way conversation is not consciously perceived, but reflexive. Importantly, cognitive influences like stress and strong emotions can alter the brain's descending feedback to the gut, affecting how the ENS functions.

**TECHNICAL
STUFF**

The ENS begins developing in the last trimester of pregnancy and continues developing after birth. This complex group of over 20 different kinds of nerves and supporting cells lives in the wall of the intestines, controlling the movement, sensory, absorptive, and secretory functions of the gut.

The main highway from the ENS to the CNS is the *vagus nerve,* the longest cranial nerve in the body. The vagus physically connects the hindbrain to the abdomen and is in charge of helping you "rest and digest." In addition, both the ENS and the CNS respond to the same neurotransmitters, including all the stress hormones. Together, these two systems are intricately involved in calming a variety of organ systems during and after the stress response.

Communication between the brain and the ENS continues during sleep. During slow-wave sleep, brain-to-gut communication slows, helping to balance the nervous system's "fight-or-flight" and "rest-and-digest" responses. This is one reason sleep is so important for mental health: Good sleep helps the brain and gut stay in healthy communication, and poor sleep throws off that connection, making gut function less stable. For more about sleep and anxious kids see Chapter 13.

Looking for clues

A medical evaluation is required for kids with CAP to distinguish an organic cause from a DGBI. Workup includes a thorough history, physical exam, and often diagnostic testing. This initial evaluation can be done by a general medical provider and doesn't require a specialist.

Gathering important clues about your child's CAP helps the evaluation process. Often, kids with CAP have patterns to their pain. Keeping a journal or notes in your phone with your child's pain frequency, timing, location, and obvious triggers or associations can be very insightful. In addition to these pain details, consider the following for additional clues:

>> New medication changes or antibiotic usage

>> Recent gastrointestinal illness or "tummy bugs"

>> Drastic changes in diet, travel history, and timing of pain

>> Family history of gut disorders

>> Recent stress or transitions

The pain patterns and associations in a child with CAP can be exceptionally variable. Normal life changes in environment, activity, stress level, and diet can make pain change. Observe what you can, but don't be too determined to find an absolute cause.

Table 6-1 is an introduction to the most common causes of CAP in kids and their treatments. If an organic cause is found, a targeted treatment plan will improve the pain. If the pain is thought to be due to a DGBI, the treatment plan focuses on reassurance, education, and symptom management.

TABLE 6-1 Common Causes of Chronic Abdominal Pain in Children

Cause	Age at Presentation	Clinical Features	Treatment
Abdominal migraine	2–10 years	Recurring abdominal pain "episodes," dull to severe pain, associated with migraine features (nausea/vomiting, pallor) but without headache	Treated like migraine, including medical management, therapy, and coping skills
Anxiety	4–11 years	Ill-defined pain around belly button, lasts less than one hour, resolves spontaneously, most common upon awakening or in the evening, triggered by stress or transitions, no pain in between episodes, associated other anxiety symptoms, unrelated to pooping or eating	Stress management, pain reduction, therapy, medical management — all the things in this book!
Carbohydrate malabsorption (for example, sucrose, fructose, lactose)	Toddler to teen	Diarrhea, bloating, gas, and/or abdominal cramping, specifically after eating dishes containing large amounts of triggering foods	Supplements, dietary changes (**Note:** Lactose intolerance is rare prior to puberty)
Constipation	Toddler to teen	After-dinner pain, night pain, low appetite, pooping during the night	See the later section "Getting the scoop on poop"
Dyspepsia	Around 10 years	Early fullness, bloating, nausea, no change in pain with pooping, increased pain after eating, frequency associated with anxiety	Smaller, frequent meals, dietary changes, behavioral modification, coping skills, limited use of medications

Cause	Age at Presentation	Clinical Features	Treatment
Gastric reflux	Toddlers to teen	Early morning pain, early fullness, nausea, chest pain, chronic cough, known family history	Antacids, medications, dietary changes, food schedule changes
Inflammatory bowel disease	Over age 2	Lower abdominal pain, increased pain after meals, pooping at night, bloody diarrhea. Anemia, mouth ulcers, slow growth, delayed puberty	GI specialist

Warning signs to never ignore

WARNING

In children with abdominal pain, there are symptoms of greater concern. These "red flags" require a medical evaluation. Call your doctor if your child is experiencing any of the following:

>> Significant vomiting (over 24 hours, signs of dehydration) or refusal to eat

>> Chronic diarrhea (more than two weeks), black tarry stool, or blood in stool

>> Unexplained fever or weight loss

>> Urinary symptoms or severe back pain

>> Unexplained rashes

Getting the scoop on poop

Of the causes of CAP, constipation rules them all. Constipation is so common in young kids that most doctors are going to assume any chronic pain symptom is due to constipation — and they are most often correct. Anxious kids are especially prone to constipation due to the stress response's effect on the gut, making it an important thing to properly identify and treat.

The crisis of constipation in kids isn't just about Goldfish crackers or too much milk. Certainly, our modern, carb-loaded, processed diets aren't helpful to gut health. But even with better nutrition and hydration, a kid's gut motility can be weird. Slower transit times in the gut can lead to chronically hard poop that's irrelevant of what they eat. Also, a typical kid's diet is erratic, not fiber-filled, and hydration is tough to track. And especially in young kids, behavioral issues and emotional factors heavily influence the ENS, changing how and when they go.

Constipation in kids is defined by incomplete evacuation of the lower colon, not the frequency or firmness of stools. Kids can have "normal" poops and still be constipated. Some kids even have runny poop or leaking accidents due to constipation.

REMEMBER

Constipation in kids can be painless, and kids with constipation can poop every day.

Management of constipation includes encouraging the complete elimination of the lower colon by whatever means necessary, and increasing muscle tone and building neurologic connections. This is often done using stool softeners, gentle laxatives, or behavioral management until the colon can respond correctly to fiber-filled foods. Then, the transition to food-based management can begin. Biofeedback, pelvic floor therapy, and progressive relaxation can also be used with kids who are motivated.

TIP

Excessive fiber is typically not the answer to kids' constipation. There is little evidence that fiber-only initiatives can help initial constipation management due to various types of fiber absorption and varied doses for effect. Talk with your doctor about what poop-enhancing solutions they prefer.

Helping tummy pain at home

For anxious kids with abdominal symptoms, the pain can be exceptionally distracting, and it increases worry about their body. Once the pain is understood and well-controlled, their anxiety will often lessen.

Here are some tips to try at home to help make tummy pain go away. The following suggestions should be used only for chronic pain symptoms without any warning signs, and preferably after a thorough medical evaluation:

>> **Manage heartburn.** Dietary changes can help heartburn symptoms, like limiting citrus fruits, spicy foods, and carbonated drinks, and avoiding late-night eating. For occasional pain, simple calcium-based antacids are available for kids and are typically safe to try according to package directions. In a pinch, a small peppermint-flavored candy can do the trick, too. If you find yourself offering these to your child most days of the week, check in with your doctor.

>> **Skip the probiotic.** Although heavily marketed for abdominal pain symptoms, current evidence shows modest, if any, effect with their use. At this time, the American Academy of Pediatrics and other child health organizations caution that probiotics are not universally effective.

>> **Avoid random food elimination diets.** Unless there is a very clear association between a specific food item and your child's symptoms, random food elimination trials are rarely helpful (like eliminating dairy or gluten). Plus, they run the risk of making a child feel like they are different or something is wrong, which is especially troubling in anxious kids.

>> **Ignore large lab panels looking for food allergies.** These tests are often misinterpreted and lead to unneeded elimination diets in an otherwise healthy child. Suspicion of food allergies in children is best guided by your pediatrician or allergist.

>> **Watch stooling habits.** A healthy kid poop looks like soft serve ice cream and happens at least once a day — never hard balls or big enough to clog the toilet. Kids shouldn't be straining when they poop; using a small stool to position themselves on the toilet with their knees higher than their hips can help. Increase water intake and offer healthy snacks. Talk with your doctor about safe stool softeners you can try.

>> **Coach deep breathing**. Deep breathing exercises stretch the diaphragm and stimulate the vagus nerve. When the vagus is triggered, the relaxation centers in the ENS light up, relieving abdominal pain. For more calming techniques see Chapter 16.

>> **Offer heat and pressure.** A heating pad and/or weighted stuffed animal can be great helpers, especially in the evening and during relaxation time.

>> **Limit late-night eating.** Our guts slow down when we sleep. In kids, this can be especially pain-triggering if there's a large amount of undigested food in their stomach when they go to bed. As your family's undoubtedly crazy schedule allows, try to have dinner earlier in the evening, and skip the milk or snack before bed.

>> **Encourage exercise.** When you get the body moving, the gut moves, too. All kids, and especially those with abdominal pain, should get their body sweaty every day through healthy movement.

>> **Go to school and activities.** Kids can go to school with chronic stomachaches and proper support. If your child has no fever, diarrhea, vomiting, sore throat, or other signs of acute illness, they need to be in the classroom. Talk with your doctor about developing a pain plan that can be assisted by the school nurse to keep your child in school as much as possible.

Managing Sleepless Nights

All kids have bad nights of sleep from time to time; it's totally normal. But when sleep is disrupted for weeks in a row, or your child's sleep habits are disrupting the whole family, it may be a primary sleep disorder. Identifying and treating these conditions improves nighttime sleep quality and daytime behavior. A sleep assessment to identify primary sleep disorders should be part of any mental health evaluation.

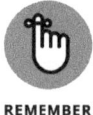

REMEMBER

The importance of sleep cannot be overstated. In fact, you can find sleep details in four different chapters of this book — more than any other anxiety-related topic. If you can make only one positive change toward mental wellness, the most impact for your effort comes from improving your family's sleep.

There's a biological reason why anxiety is worse at night. As you fall asleep, your brain powers down in stages. The thinking brain slows down first, diminishing logical reasoning. Meanwhile, the emotional brain remains active, heightening emotional experiences. This sleepy imbalance makes it harder to rationalize and manage anxious thoughts as you drift off.

Surveying slumbering symptoms

More than half of all kids experience some type of sleep issue during childhood, but only about 4 percent are diagnosed with a primary sleep disorder. Most common childhood sleep problems can be identified through careful observation and conversation with your child's primary care doctor. If issues continue, formal diagnostic testing by a pediatric sleep medicine specialist may be recommended.

Sleep problems are common in anxious kids, but a primary sleep disorder can make the daytime symptoms exponentially worse. Table 6-2 can help you determine whether your anxious kid needs a formal sleep evaluation.

TABLE 6-2 ## Common Childhood Sleep Disorders

Sleep Disorder	Characteristics	Clinical Features	Treatment
Behavioral insomnia	10–30% of kids; the most common sleep disorder in anxious kids	Sleep-onset or limit-setting challenges, leads to a learned inability to fall asleep or stay asleep alone	Prevention, parent education (find tips in Chapter 17)
Confusional arousal: partial arousal that occurs between deep sleep and wakefulness	3–13 years; positive family history	"Sleep drunk," slowed responsiveness, slurred speech, confusion with awakening; first third of sleep; 5–30 minutes; no sweating, agitation, or increased heart rate	Usually resolves on its own; scheduled awakenings; keep safe, leave alone

(continued)

TABLE 6-2 *(continued)*

Sleep Disorder	Characteristics	Clinical Features	Treatment
Obstructive sleep apnea (OSA): upper airway obstruction that disrupts normal sleep patterns	Onset between 2–8 years, when tonsils rapidly grow	Loud snoring more than three nights a week, unusual sleep positions, morning headache, daytime behavior changes, enlarged tonsils or adenoids, sunken chest, small jaw	Tonsillectomy; CPAP; nasal steroids
Restless leg syndrome (RLS) and periodic limb movement disorder (PLMD): limb movements during sleep associated with sleep disruption	2% of kids; most common in females; strong family history	Negative behavior and mood, associated with ADHD, may be associated with iron deficiency, triggered by heavy exercise	Iron replacement; remove possible triggers
Sleep terror: crying out in perceived intense fear, though not awake	1–5 percent of kids; early childhood onset; peak incidence is 5–7 years	Perceived intense fear, occurs in first third of sleep duration, rapid return to sleep, physical symptoms — flushed, sweaty, rapid heart rate, no memory of event in the morning	Leave undisturbed, most become more agitated with calming; scheduled awakenings; most resolve by age 12
Sleepwalking: walking during sleep, eyes open, difficult to awaken	More common in males; onset between 8–12 years; strong family history; 15% of kids; typically gone by puberty	Confusion, rapid return to sleep, typically in the first third of the night's sleep, lasts 5–15 minutes, often occurs during illness or in new environments	Usually resolves on its own; bedroom/home safety; scheduled awakenings

Getting better zzz's

For all the worried kids out there who have trouble sleeping, here are some safe things to try at home:

» **Determine family sleep goals.** From day one of parenthood, talk with your partner about how you want to prioritize and protect family sleep. Choose realistic expectations and boundaries, practice great sleep hygiene, and keep sleeping spaces electronics-free. Start the habits early to avoid the need for behavioral intervention in the future. For more about optimizing sleep see Chapter 13.

>> **Manage other conditions.** Be sure to properly manage chronic medical conditions known to disrupt sleep, such as asthma, concussion, gastric reflux, chronic pain, and attention-deficit/hyperactivity disorder (ADHD).

TIP

Sleep science in kids is rapidly expanding, and there are many other causes of sleep disruption in kids. If you're worried about something you observe during your child's sleep, grab video if you can, and visit your doctor.

>> **Visit the dentist.** The mouth can show evidence of conditions like gastric reflux, OSA, and teeth grinding. Every child should see the dentist twice a year, beginning in toddlerhood. During your child's appointment, ask the dentist whether they notice signs of concern.

>> **Add iron.** Iron deficiency is associated with decreased sleep quality. Sleep physicians often check iron levels and recommend supplements, if a child is deficient. Talk to your doctor if you're interested in exploring this as an option. For more about iron and anxiety see Chapter 11.

TIP

Some researchers believe that the pain commonly attributed to "growing pains" is an expression of RLS. If your child routinely gets growing pains, talk to your doc about RLS as a possibility.

>> **Skip the wearables.** Sleep tracking devices are available for babies and children. Although a tempting way to watch sleep quality, these devices haven't been standardized to provide practically usable data about a child's sleep. Plus, wearables for kids and other tech trackers have been known to increase parental anxiety. And nobody needs more of that.

TIP

If you're trying any intervention for sleep improvement, keep a diary of progress. It's the only way to keep an accurate record of trends and patterns. Include naps, eating habits, notable activity in the day, and sleep/wake times.

Dealing with Nagging Headaches

Headaches are a common symptom of many illnesses, some chronic conditions, or unavoidable changes in our environment. In addition, headaches have an intricate and complicated relationship with our mood.

Due to the complex relationship between stress, emotions, and pain, headaches in children with anxiety are harder to treat. It's not clear if these kids have a more stressful life, or if they are more sensitive to stress. Regardless, untreated headaches can be exceptionally interruptive to a child's day, cause problems with school absenteeism, reduce focus, and interfere with making friends. Correctly diagnosing and identifying a headache cause can help kids thrive.

REMEMBER

Headaches can cause anxiety, and anxiety can cause headaches.

Warning signs to never ignore

WARNING

Some characteristics and associated symptoms in kids with headaches deserve a visit to a qualified health professional. Call the doctor now if your child is experiencing any of the following:

>> The worst or first headache your child has experienced

>> Recent head trauma, such as a fall or sports injury

>> Vision changes, repeated vomiting, or fever

>> Inability to walk, talk, or eat normally

>> Pain that wakes them from sleep or occurs in the early morning

>> Known sickle cell disease

>> Chronic and progressive (getting worse over time) headaches

Distinguishing headache types

There are two general headache types in kids: tension headaches and migraines. The following sections walk you through the differences.

TIP

If your child experiences headaches, keep a diary. Note your child's headache location, severity, timing, and associated factors or symptoms. When asking kids about their symptoms, ask open-ended questions to get the best information.

Troubling tension headaches

Tension type headaches are the most common. These are called "hat band headaches" because that is where the pain is located on the head. Although the exact mechanism isn't understood, tension headaches are thought to be caused by physical stress or bad posture, dehydration and hunger, genetic predisposition, or neurologic sensitivity.

When kids have tension headaches, their pain is difficult but not incapacitating. Although they are not fully themselves, the pain is not severe enough to limit a child's ability to go to school, attend activities, or play their favorite sport. This is quite different than the pain level and change of behavior that kids with migraine experience.

TIP

Every parent of a kid with head pain is worried about a brain tumor. This is rarely the case. But don't sit alone in your worry! Visit your child's doctor to get you on the right track.

Menacing migraines

Headaches due to migraine are less common, with about 5 percent of kids experiencing migraine before the age of 10. The cause of migraine headaches is complex and currently believed to be due to primary brain cell dysfunction that leads to increased sensitivity to a variety of genetic and environmental factors. It's also thought that certain neurotransmitters, including serotonin, play a role in migraine. To find out more about serotonin see Chapter 2.

Migraine looks different in kids than in adults. In kids, the headache is typically preceded by irritability, fatigue, or behavioral changes up to a day prior to the headache onset. The headache is often on both sides of the head and doesn't last long. The headache is severe and often associated with vomiting and sensitivity to bright lights and loud sounds. These kids stop what they are doing and need to go to a dark room and lie down. After the event, they are exhausted.

Headaches due to migraine are more common in kids with internalizing disorders, especially anxiety. Migraine is also associated in kids with a history of paroxysmal vertigo (brief periods of dizziness or spinning that self-resolve), benign intermittent torticollis (recurring neck spasms that cause the head to tilt), colic, motion sickness, and CAP.

TIP

Unique to kids is a condition called abdominal migraine. Refer to Table 6-1 for details.

Relieving headaches at home

Treating headaches improves anxiety, and treating anxiety improves headaches. The following list includes simple and effective headache management tips that help anxious kids. For kids with persisting symptoms, your child's doctor may suggest evidence-based therapeutics or anti-anxiety medication to bolster pain tolerance, support neurotransmitter function, and lead to more headache-free days.

>> **Prioritize healthy basics.** Basics always come first. Routine sleep, daily exercise, balanced nutrition, and quality sleep help the whole family, including any child with headaches.

>> **Watch the screen time.** Studies have suggested a relationship between screen exposure and headaches. Healthy management of educational and non-educational screen time, hydration, sitting posture, and taking frequent screen breaks may decrease this risk. For more on managing screen time in anxious kids see Chapter 13.

>> **Consider eating frequency.** Try to avoid prolonged fasting. Offer a daily breakfast and additional small snacks throughout the day.

>> **Use pain reducers**. Over-the-counter pain medication, like ibuprofen, is safe and effective to give young children for headaches. Dose by your child's weight, using the information on the packaging, and follow the recommended frequency. If you're using over-the-counter pain reliever more than a few times per week, check in with your doctor.

Never offer aspirin to children for pain or fever due to its association with Reye syndrome.

>> **Shop supplements.** There's moderate evidence to support using nutritional supplements for headache prevention. Headache prevention plans may include daily weight-based doses of magnesium, riboflavin, CoQ10, or an omega-3 fatty acid blend. For more on supplements see Chapter 11.

>> **Continue activities or situations that may cause a tension headache.** Don't avoid activities that may cause a mild headache. Over time, this accommodation behavior will teach your child that they don't have the capacity or power to overcome the pain on their own.

>> **Resist turning your life upside down looking for "triggers."** Kids' bodies are rapidly changing, and the triggers are, too. Some families spend so much time looking for the cause that they don't properly care for the headache happening today. At the most basic level, headaches just mean a bad day. And we all have bad days.

TIP

There's little evidence that vision problems are a primary cause of headaches in kids. However, most preventative care guidelines suggest all children should get a comprehensive eye examination by an eye professional (not just a school or office-based vision screen) after the age of 3. If your child hasn't had a comprehensive eye exam, consider scheduling one.

Experiencing Urinary Issues

Kids with anxiety often experience changes in bathroom habits, especially at school. Interestingly, some kids with anxiety use the bathroom more, some less. These behavior changes often serve as clues to shifts in a child's mood at school and at home.

For example, Ray, a healthy 10-year-old girl, came to my office after her teacher complained that she was going to the bathroom too much. Here is her story:

> Ray says she feels an urgent need to use the bathroom every 20–30 minutes at school, even though she often passes only small amounts of urine each time. This issue doesn't happen as frequently at home on weekends. Ray doesn't report pain, burning, or other symptoms of a urinary tract infection, but her mom is worried about an infection. When her urine test is normal, more questions get to the root of Ray's problem.

Ray was experiencing frequent urination due to anxiety. More questions revealed that she was recently experiencing more stress from peer challenges at school. With the school counselor's help, managing Ray's stress led to a decrease in her need to go to the bathroom during the day.

TIP

Sometimes anxious kids ask to go to the bathroom just to get a break from a stressful situation in the classroom, or as an avoidance behavior. Teachers can't always tell whether frequent restroom use signals a physical or mental health issue, but in either case, it's an important clue that something needs attention.

The stress response stimulates the sympathetic nervous system. During times of fear or anxiety, there is increasing muscle tension in the body, including the pelvic floor and bladder. This causes problems with storing urine (pee accidents or frequency), voiding behaviors (hesitancy, difficulty peeing or straining), or post-voiding leakage (pee dribbles and incomplete emptying). These symptoms are exceptionally disruptive at school if kids feel like they need to pee all the time. And the stress of possibly having an accident also increases anxiety — a vicious cycle!

Peeing too much

For kids who pee too much, visit the doctor to ensure that your child doesn't have an infection or other treatable issue. If your child's medical evaluation is all clear, here are some things to help limit bathroom breaks:

- » **Control constipation.** Constipation can cause bladder pressure, decreasing the amount of pee the bladder can hold. Treating constipation can improve urinary frequency by giving the bladder more space to relax.

- » **Schedule voiding.** Using a "potty watch" or timing device lets your child know the next time they should use the restroom. Start every two hours, increasing the duration between visits over time. This form of bladder retraining can quickly improve symptoms; talk with your doctor for details.

- » **Avoid electronics in the bathroom.** A special activity book or reading material can help a child relax, but screens don't belong in the bathroom. (For adults, too!)

- » **Watch liquid intake.** Avoid drinks with caffeine, bubbles, or juice or sports drinks that may irritate the bladder or cause extra urine.

- » **Stay clean and comfy.** Choose clothing, bedding, and other products that are comfortable but also encourage proper hygiene.

- » **Connect with professionals.** If your child isn't showing signs of progress, connecting with a pediatric pelvic floor or behavioral therapist can be helpful. Rarely, medication is used with the guidance of a urinary specialist.

REMEMBER

Keep in mind that kids aren't going to the bathroom to intentionally be disruptive or defiant. They are responding to their body's signal that they need to go. Provide emotional support and understanding to decrease stress while re-training their body's signaling.

TECHNICAL STUFF

Pollakiuria is the medical term for frequent urination during times of stress or anxiety. It's also an impressive, 17-point Scrabble word.

Peeing too little

For some kids, the act of peeing can be anxiety-provoking. For example, kids with "shy bladder syndrome," which is a form of social anxiety, cannot pee in front of others or use public bathrooms. As a result, these kids have behavior changes, like looking distracted or inattentive when they are focusing on repressing the need to go. Other kids drastically decrease their fluid intake to suppress the urge. These changes can lead to additional problems like constipation or urinary tract infections.

REMEMBER

The school restroom can be a scary place. Kids choose bathroom avoidance due to significant social issues, like bullying that takes place or feeling that they are unsafe. The bathroom environment can be unclean, without proper supplies or properly locking doors. They may be uncomfortable with their body making sounds or smells that would be embarrassing. These are all issues that can lead to unhealthy voiding and stooling behaviors at school.

For kids who use the restroom on a less frequent basis, many of the techniques used for kids who pee too much will also help (see the previous section). Things like scheduled voiding practice and watching constipation can improve symptoms. However, since urine holding is a form of social anxiety, most kids need expert-guided therapy to decrease their fear of urinating in public places. Talk with your doctor for suggestions.

Handling Concerning Chest Pain

When a child complains of chest pain, it's common (and normal!) for parents to panic. They often fear that their child is having a heart attack, has a significant illness, or is at risk for sudden death. Thankfully, these are exceptionally rare causes of chest pain in kids. The most common cause? You guessed it — anxiety.

REMEMBER

Unlike adults, most chest pain in children is typically not associated with any serious medical conditions. Understanding the cause of pain and working toward solutions will lead to fewer stressful or anxious days.

Reacting to stress

Anxiety accounts for about 30 percent of chest pain in children. That's a lot. Chest pain in kids is often associated with significant stressful events or life changes. Most children with psychiatric chest pain also have other somatic complaints like headache or abdominal pain, and many also have sleep disruption. When the anxiety is treated, chest pain is relieved. Chest pain is also a common symptom of panic attacks. For more details about panic disorder see Chapter 16.

Chest pain from anxiety is thought to be caused by the stress response. During stress, the blood pressure and heart rate rise when the sympathetic nervous system is activated. This can lead to sweating, hyperventilation, and dull, achy pain. Anxiety can also cause muscle spasms that can feel like chest pain or tightness.

Chest pain is associated with school absenteeism and restriction from sports and other activities for fear of cardiac cause. The reality is that the vast, vast majority of healthy children who complain of chest pain don't have a life-threatening condition and should continue to participate in school and sports. Chest pain in children is common and treatable, and rarely requires extensive testing.

TIP

Chest pain can be caused by carrying a heavy backpack on one shoulder. Teach your kids to carry backpacks with both straps.

Warning signs to never ignore

WARNING

Concerning chest pain in children doesn't happen in isolation. Of the 5 percent of children who have a life-threatening reason for chest pain, associated symptoms are also present. In other words, these kids look sick. Here are some red flags to look out for:

>> Pain during physical activity or exercise that is bad enough to make them stop

>> Pain that worsens over a few hours

>> Pain with other symptoms, such as difficulty breathing, fever, vomiting, dizziness, or fainting

>> Pain with rapid heart rate or sweating

>> Pain in a child with a family history of heart issues or unexplained early death

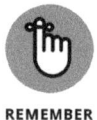

Children with chest pain and a personal history of heart disease or with high-risk genetic syndromes, connective tissue disorders, sickle cell disease, or a family history of early-onset heart disease need to promptly call their doctor for evaluation.

Taking Care of Tics (Not Ticks)

Tics are a common movement disorder. Ticks are infection-ridden, blood-sucking bugs. I'm not talking about bugs.

Tics are a form of neurodevelopment disorder, characterized by repetitive, recognizable, unwanted movements or vocalizations. Tics nearly always begin in childhood, with up to 10 percent of normal, healthy children experiencing a tic at some point during the childhood years. Tics are also commonly seen in anxious kids. Estimates vary, but about 30 percent of children who tic have anxiety.

Not all kids with tics have anxiety, but many kids with anxiety have tics.

Think your kid is ticcing? Grab your phone and capture some video. Your pediatrician will help to determine whether what you're observing is a tic, another type of movement disorder, or part of normal child development.

Tics don't happen during sleep. If your child is having repetitive movements or vocalizations during sleep, take a video and visit your pediatrician.

Identifying tics

Tics are distinguishable from other movement disorders by a few characteristics, such as involving the head and upper body, and being discrete and nonrhythmic. Interestingly, tics change over time, with each individual often developing a unique combination of a few different tics. Some of the most common tics in childhood include the following:

>> Blinking, squinting, or wide opening of eyes

>> Nose twitching

- » Head or neck jerking
- » Arm, hand, or shoulder movements
- » Throat clearing or tongue clicking
- » Grunting, sniffing, humming, or word repetition

Tics typically start between ages 3 and 9 and are most severe between ages 9 and 11. *Transient tics* stop within a few months and rarely require treatment. However, current evidence suggests that *provisional tics* may last longer, especially in children with anxiety or other behavioral disorders.

Managing tics

Most children with tic disorders don't need professional help. However, if you notice your child ticcing, the following are ways to support them at home:

- » **Create an understanding and supportive home environment.** Avoid reacting to your child's tic to limit frustration. Anticipate times and environments where ticcing may increase, but don't avoid those situations. Anticipate increased ticcing after school if your child is suppressing movements during school hours.

  Kids who tic need school support. One of the best things you can do for a child with a tic disorder is get support at school. Be open with your child's teacher, offer information about the disorder, and advocate for your child to have extra physical activity to help release the tics.

- » **Learn neurofeedback techniques.** There is a strong emotional component to ticcing. Tics can increase from stress, birthdays, holidays, going back to school, or talking or thinking about tics. Tics decrease during deep concentration. Stress reduction using neurofeedback, imagery training, and relaxation techniques has been shown to be potentially helpful to decrease tic frequency.

- » **Sleep!** Studies have suggested that sleep loss and fatigue increase ticcing. However, many children with tic disorders also experience worsened sleep efficiency and parasomnias, such as sleepwalking and night terrors. If sleep problems improve and sleep is more efficient, tics tend to improve.

>> **Work out.** Exercise has been shown to decrease ticcing both during the exercise and in the period following. Exercise is also shown to decrease anxiety in children with tic disorders. For more on the power of exercise and anxiety see Chapter 13.

When a child's tics cause social embarrassment or physical discomfort, or interfere with daily life or activities, they need more aggressive treatment. Behavioral intervention therapy is the primary treatment, although it can be hard to find these specialized therapists. Online and app-based programs are available. See the Appendix for details. There are medications to help ticcing if behavioral support fails.

TIP

Most children with tics don't need specialized treatment. However, if your child's tics last longer than one year, interfere with school performance, or cause social disruption, connect with your pediatrician for professional help.

EXAMINING PANDAS/PANS

In the early 1990s, researchers reported a group of young children who developed severe tic symptoms after a Group A streptococcal (GAS) infection. As more children presented with sudden-onset neuropsychiatric issues following GAS infections, researchers began investigating a potential link. They proposed an autoimmune process triggered by strep infections as a possible cause of severe movement disorders, known as PANDAS (Pediatric Autoimmune Neuropsychiatric Disorders Associated with Streptococcal infections).

As research has progressed, PANDAS is now thought to represent a subset of a larger spectrum of acute-onset neuropsychiatric symptoms. In turn, the American Academy of Pediatrics currently refers to this condition as PANS (Pediatric Acute-Onset Neuropsychiatric Syndrome). The cause of PANS is unknown, but it appears to be associated with both infectious and non-infectious conditions.

Children with suspected PANS experience a sudden, dramatic onset of obsessive-compulsive behaviors, often accompanied by anxiety, tics, food restriction, developmental regression, irritability, and/or sensory abnormalities. Current treatments focus on each child's unique spectrum of symptoms.

Concerned pediatric experts are still learning more about this rare syndrome. Since the risk factors, diagnostic markers, and biological mechanisms of PANS remain unclear, getting a definitive diagnosis remains challenging. Meanwhile, the lack of clear guidance has made families who believe their child has PANS feel very isolated and alone.

If you observe a sharp increase in your child's anxiety after an illness, talk with your doctor. For most children, the brief rise will naturally regress without intervention. If additional testing or treatment needs to be considered, your doctor can help.

Watching Out for Thyroid Disorders

The thyroid is a small, butterfly-shaped gland that lives in the front of the neck, near the voice box. As part of the endocrine system, the thyroid's primary job is to produce thyroid hormones. In kids, thyroid hormones have a major role in brain maturation, body growth, and metabolism, and are vital to maintain many important body functions.

When the thyroid produces too much or too little thyroid hormone, the effects can be seen in a variety of ways. Generally speaking, too much hormone speeds up the body's metabolism and too little slows it down.

In children with thyroid disease, hypothyroidism is more common. Low thyroid levels are associated with certain genetic and autoimmune conditions, such as Down syndrome, celiac disease, type 1 diabetes, and Turner syndrome. Children with these conditions should have routine screening for thyroid health.

Excessive thyroid hormone can significantly affect mood, often causing anxiety symptoms. Hyperthyroidism most commonly affects genetic females, often appearing around puberty, though it can impact kids of any age. Because thyroid hormone plays a crucial role in brain function, mental health changes from thyroid disease can appear months before physical symptoms. Once abnormal thyroid levels are identified and normalized, anxiety tends to improve.

TIP

If there is a strong family history of thyroid issues in your family, talk with your doctors about routinely screening your child's thyroid levels. A simple blood test may be able to detect a change before serious symptoms begin.

2

Diagnosing Child Anxiety

Understand the process of diagnosing a child anxiety disorder, starting with a visit to the pediatrician. Prepare for the doctor visit by gathering history, asking for teacher feedback, and sharing organized family history to make the appointment more productive. Determine the important questions to ask a child's healthcare provider.

Discover ways parents can help a child fully participate during the office visit, especially if they are anxious. Understand confidentiality as a part of a child's medical visit and what to expect — including a helpful list of doctor office "don'ts" for any type of medical visit.

Recognize that a child's symptoms don't clearly lead to an anxiety diagnosis. Look into the psychological evaluation, including what type of experts can diagnose child anxiety, what the evaluation entails, and how a child will participate. Be aware of alternative diagnoses that may present with anxiety-like behaviors.

Chapter **7**

Visiting the Doctor

I f you're concerned that your child has an anxiety disorder, one of the first places to turn is your child's pediatrician. A visit to the doctor helps define the issues your child is facing, work toward a proper diagnosis, and develop an appropriate plan for your family. Most importantly, visiting the doctor establishes a working partnership focused entirely on your child's physical and mental wellness.

The challenge is that most people — especially kids — don't like to go to the doctor's office. It's filled with unknowns, new people, strange equipment, and things that hurt. I know the doctor's office can be a scary place; I work in one. I also know there are lots of ways to make the visit more effective and pleasant for everyone.

In this chapter, you discover how to find the right pediatrician for your family. Once that person is found, I teach you the best ways to make the doctor visit efficient and effective. Finally, I offer pediatrician-proven tips for a successful visit day.

Finding a Great Pediatrician

First things first, you need a great pediatrician. I hope you already have one. If you don't, let me help guide your search. The availability of pediatricians and other primary care providers for kids varies widely across the United States and around the world. Ultimately, you're looking for an accessible, qualified, compatible partner in the care of your children.

TIP

Most primary care providers look alike on paper. It's hard to tell from a Google search or generic website who is going to be the best match for your family. Personal recommendations are a great place to start. Ask friends, family, neighbors, and co-workers where they take their kids for care to help start your search.

Once you have a few names, check out the basics. A great pediatrician should have a website with office hours and locations, contact numbers, hospital affiliations, credentials, and essential biographical information. Connect with the office to ensure that the provider is taking new patients and accepts your insurance. For most families, a strong personal recommendation from a friend and a quick insurance check are all that's needed to press forward and make the first appointment.

TIP

All pediatricians have completed medical school and residency, passed certification exams, and have years of experience working with kids. What you're looking for is someone who's welcoming and likable. Not sure? Schedule an interview to find out. Most providers welcome the opportunity to connect with prospective parents in person or on the phone to see whether the partnership is going to be a good fit. The following are some questions to ask during a physician interview:

>> **"Tell me about your office."** Use the web to get the basics, but ask this question to let the doctor tell you where their office shines. Hours and accessibility? Length of appointment times? Special offers?

>> **"Why did you choose to be a pediatrician?"** The million-dollar question. Of all the medical specialties, why did they choose to take care of kids?

» **"I'm concerned about [insert concern here]. How do you help families like mine?"** Sharing a bit of your child's history or current concern can help you get a taste of how your family's needs will be supported. This question will also tap into accessibility. Especially for kids with mental health issues, you'll likely be seeing the doctor multiple times per year. Does this provider have the space to see your child routinely?

» **"What do you love about your job?"** Do they have a passion for a certain type of patient or have special training in a certain area? Do they love to teach? Is this someone you can have a great conversation with?

» **"What do you do outside of work?"** Asking the doctor what they enjoy doing outside of work may spark a personal connection or common interest that ensures that they will be the best partner for your family's care.

» **"How do you feel about vaccinations and antibiotics?"** It's important to understand how a provider is going to educate and support your family during medical decision-making. This question gives you an opportunity to hear how the physician will share their expertise about important medical inventions, as well as allow you to share your own concerns or beliefs.

Preparing for the Office Visit

Once you have selected your child's doctor or made an appointment with your existing pediatrician, it's time to prepare yourself and your child for the office visit. Spending time collecting your child's history and your concerns will make the visit more efficient and collaborative.

Organizing and prioritizing

The doctor's office is an inherently busy place. Trust me when I say that we have the mutual goal of getting as much accomplished for your child during the visit as we can. To do that efficiently, we need your help. Thoughtfully preparing for your office visit is one way to ensure that it will meet your expectations and be helpful to your child.

>> **Start from the beginning.** When did you first notice the symptoms? What did you notice first? Have the symptoms changed over time? How are things the same or different? Why are you coming to the doctor for this *now?* How have things been in the last two weeks?

TIP

>> **Sketch a symptom timeline.** Mental and physical health diagnoses are often defined by the duration of time. Knowing rough start and stop dates of symptoms can be helpful.

>> **Describe your concerns and observations with specific details.** Saying your child is "acting up," "has big emotions," or "doesn't act like other kids" may be true statements, but these comments aren't helpful to determine a diagnosis or treatment goals. Choose specific behaviors or observations that brought you to the office.

>> **Define your primary concern.** If your doctor had a magic wand and could improve one thing, what would that one thing be? That's your primary concern. It's important to define your primary concern because kids often have more than one thing going on, especially with the mental and physical symptoms of anxiety. Identifying and sharing your primary concern will help determine next steps and create a benchmark to monitor improvement.

>> **Create your goals and questions based on your primary concern.** Make your list. Check it twice. Bring a notebook full of questions or have a list on your phone to organize the conversation and ensure that your top-level questions will be answered. In turn, it helps the doctor to know what is most important to you.

>> **Collect videos of behaviors.** Watching how your child moves or behaves in real time can be helpful, if needed.

>> **List any prior treatments, therapy, medications, or supplements.** Knowing which prior treatments have worked and failed can be great diagnostic clues.

>> **Gather any significant personal or family history.** Include both mental and physical conditions that run in the family.

>> **Prepare to share major life events, transitions, or changes that have occurred since the onset of your child's behaviors.** Kids often show temporary behavior changes after major life events like a move, divorce, or loss. Recognizing these triggers can shape a diagnosis and guide treatment.

Engaging educators

Educators are vital health historians for our kids. Children spend most of their awake hours with their teachers, whose input on observations and patterns can be exceptionally helpful for all sorts of physical and mental health diagnoses. In addition, educators can be valuable advocates for their students by bringing new behaviors or symptoms to a parent's attention.

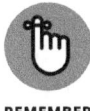

REMEMBER

If a teacher shares a behavioral concern about your child, take it seriously. It takes a village, and educators are there to fully support the health and wellness of all of their students.

Some childhood mental health diagnoses require feedback from an educator. Let your child's teacher know that you're visiting the doctor and may be looking for their observations in the classroom. This gives them some time to complete any formal intake forms, prepare email comments, or plan for conversations during parent-teacher conferences. For some kids, valuable feedback can also be gained from coaches, music instructors, leadership at religious centers, former or current therapists, or after-school care providers.

TIP

If your child already holds a 504 plan or Individualized Educational Program (IEP), a copy of that document can often be helpful to the provider. Bring it with you to the office visit. To find out about educational support plans for children with anxiety see Chapter 14.

Including all caregivers

There are all types of families and all types of caregiving arrangements. Healthcare providers who work with kids are very familiar with making accommodations so that all family members are equally available to participate in a child's care. All you need to do is let them know!

As able, all of your child's significant caregivers should participate in the initial medical visit. If all caregivers cannot be present, grab your phone. With permission, your child's other caregivers can join by FaceTime, conference call, or secure telehealth service. Alternatively, doctors welcome written communication from other caregivers. See Chapter 17 for more insight into co-parenting a child with anxiety.

Asking for a private conversation

It's not uncommon for families to ask to speak with me privately about a child's behavior. Parents don't want to "talk bad" in front of their kid or make their child feel shameful about a situation. Talking privately allows parents to offer their honest observations and feelings about a child's behavior and gives them an opportunity to disclose important details about a situation that their child may be unaware of.

I am careful to avoid private parent conversations when young kids are in the office. Kids are smart, and they know when parents are talking "behind their back." When a secret conversation is with a doctor, kids worry that something is wrong with them or that something bad is going to happen — especially anxious kids! If a child feels stress from separation or is worrying about the content of a private discussion, my ability to build a trusted relationship with my patient becomes more difficult.

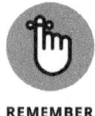

REMEMBER

The patient in the room is your child. A great pediatrician is going to prioritize the comfort, care, and safety of the child in the room. Always.

TIP

As much as possible, encourage your child to discuss their concerns directly with the doctor. Even young kids can offer valuable context about their behaviors, and pediatricians are skilled in having these conversations with them. If there's sensitive or safety-related information to share privately, let the doctor know in advance. This allows us to plan time at the start or end of the visit for a quick chat. Alternatively, you can send a letter or email with your concerns before the appointment.

Preparing your child

After your thoughts and questions are in order, it's helpful to prepare the patient. Great pediatricians want your child to be as comfortable as possible throughout their visit. These simple preparation steps can help them accomplish that goal:

1. **Tell your child about the appointment.**

   Doctor visits shouldn't be a surprise. Before the visit day, let your child know about the upcoming appointment and what it's for. Is this a routine physical day? A visit for stomachaches? A brain and body check? Give your child some context for the visit, allowing them the opportunity to form their own questions or share concerns.

2. **Manage expectations.**

   To the best of your knowledge, describe what will happen before, during, and after the visit. Most visits will include checking in, gathering vital signs, performing a physical exam, and lots of talking. For little kids, walking through a doctor's visit using books or videos with favorite characters can be helpful. For older kids, suggest ways that they can participate, including helping during check-in or preparing their own list of questions for the doctor.

3. **The night before, prioritize a good night's sleep.**

TIP

   Pack a snack and water bottle. Visits can be boring for a kid, so prepare the essentials to keep your child occupied. Things like coloring books, card games, electronics with headphones, and homework can help pass the time.

4. **Never promise "no shots."**

WARNING

   Kids don't like shots. I know. But promising "no shots" is a trap that makes getting shots even worse. Even though the "no shot" promise may feel like a way to reassure your child about a doctor visit, the promise is an *accommodation behavior* — an action taken by a parent to avoid their child's anxiety. Accommodation behaviors actually *increase* anxiety in anxious people because they prevent an opportunity for the anxious person to gain resiliency through facing fear. In the doctor's office, accommodation behaviors amplify your child's perception of discomfort, making getting shots more anxiety-provoking and increasing the perception of pain when administered. For ways to support kids with needle phobia see Chapter 18.

Understanding Confidentiality

REMEMBER

All medical visits are bound by confidentiality. Kids have confidentiality, too. Protecting the privacy of a child's health information is unique because it involves a minor child and their adult parents or guardians. Here is how confidentiality works in this context:

>> **Parents are directly involved during most pediatric visits.** Confidentiality is generally shared with parents because they are directly responsible for making medical decisions for their child. Doctors can discuss health concerns, diagnoses, and treatments with parents without restriction, as long as it's in the best interest of the child.

>> **Kids can talk to their doctor in private.** This is typically done closer to adolescence, but I've had situations when younger kids were able to speak more comfortably without their parents in the room. When a child speaks privately to a healthcare provider, the provider is legally bound to maintain confidentiality.

>> **Providers are legally bound to maintain confidentiality except in situations where the child is in direct harm, engaging in behavior that can seriously harm their health, or there is a risk of harm to others.** In these rare instances, doctors are required to disclose the situation to the parents and/or authorities, depending on the severity or nature of the risk.

An inherent level of mutual trust exists when a child talks with a medical provider privately. Initially, this private time makes many parents uncomfortable, which is understandable. Parents think kids are going to disclose family secrets or share something terrible. This is rarely the case.

Private discussion time between a child and a trusted healthcare provider can be an essential relationship-building tool. Most of the time, we're talking about a cool cartoon, their favorite sports team, or what they had for lunch. This discussion time is for them to share, not for me to pry. I want all of my patients to know that I'm on their side, listening, and here to help.

If a child shares something important during a private conversation, I'll always ask if I can share that with their parent. Ninety-nine percent of the time, they say yes. In those cases, I'll bring the parent back into the room and share the information with the patient present. This allows me to both fully inform the parent about the nature of the problem and keep the patient's trust.

It takes a leap of faith for parents to allow their children to talk to a healthcare provider alone. Great pediatricians respect parents for allowing this privilege and use the time to build healthy, long-term relationships with their patients and families.

Optimizing Your Appointment Day

The doctor's office can be an intimidating, busy place. And as much as we try to have each day run smoothly, some days are simply more chaotic than others. Here are some tips on getting a great start at the office:

>> **Choose a good time.** As you're able, schedule the office visit at a time when your child will be most engaged. For young kids, this means avoiding appointments during nap

time. For school-aged kids, choose appointments before or after school.

TIP

Frustrated the doctor is running late? We are, too. If your waiting time is a concern, know that most doctors are going to be running on time first thing in the morning and right after lunch.

» **Arrive early.** Allow a few moments for your child to get comfortable in the room and get to know the environment, while you have time to complete any paperwork or last-minute tasks.

TIP

» **Let your technology help, after you get consent.** Most jurisdictions will allow audio recording of medical visits. Share with your doctor that you'd like to record the visit. Once the doctor consents, this audio can be helpful to review details later or share with another caregiver.

» **Share your goals.** "The goal of my visit today is . . ." is a perfect statement that communicates your expectations to a busy doctor and can guide the conversation. Your goal can be information gathering, connecting with specialists, finding diagnostic information, determining a treatment plan, or something else.

» **Get through your list.** Tell the doc how many questions you have and start with the most important question *first.* This helps the doctor guide how to spend their time, creates expectations, and develops a follow-up framework.

» **Jot down the name of any new diagnoses, medicines, treatments, or tests**. Also write down any new instructions your provider gives you for your child.

» **Ask until you understand.** Ask your doctor about every new medicine or treatment that is prescribed and how it will help your child. Be clear about possible side effects of any intervention. If your doctor wants to run tests, ask why a test or procedure is recommended and what the results can mean. In turn, know what to expect if your child doesn't take the medicine or have the test or procedure. Ask whether your child's condition can be treated in other ways, and the pros and cons of alternative options.

>> **Schedule a follow-up visit.** Write down the time, date, and purpose. What are the goals your child is trying to reach? How are these goals going to be evaluated during the follow-up?

>> **Know how you can contact your child's provider after office hours.** This is important if your child becomes ill and you have questions or need advice.

Avoiding "Doctor Office Don'ts"

All parents want to lovingly support their child through any medical visit. In my experience, some of the most helpful and important things that support kids are what you *don't* do. The following list explains what I mean:

>> **Don't lie.** All kids deserve honesty, especially when it comes to their own body. I understand why parents may lie about an office visit — they love their kids and want to protect them from harm. But lying about why you're visiting the doctor, or about what may happen during the visit, undermines your ability to provide effective support and puts cracks in the foundation of your child's trust.

>> **Don't underestimate your child.** Kids can do amazing things, even at the doctor's office. They can explain problems, share facts, show bravery, and choose the harder path. Provide support, let them know that they can do it on their own, and prepare to be amazed!

>> **Don't threaten with pain.** If you're trying to raise an emotionally healthy child, threats of any kind are an ineffective and inappropriate form of discipline. Threats teach fear and complicity, not valuable reasoning, and don't allow a child to develop internal motivation to make better choices. In the medical office, when I overhear frustrated parents threaten "a shot" as a consequence for undesired behavior, I worry that this useless discipline strategy will erode the trust and emotional safety that I know every parent desires. For effective behavior management strategies for anxious kids see Chapter 15.

>> **Don't call the doctor or nurse the "bad guy."** I really, really hate it when a parent describes me, or my nurse, as an enemy. When a parent calls me "the bad guy," often in reference to recommending a vaccine or blood test, it creates an inherent "good versus bad" narrative in a child's imaginative mind. Don't go there. Doctors and nurses are helpers. Always.

>> **Don't talk for your child.** Pediatricians are trained to talk to kids. We want to know how they feel, what they think, and why they are worried. We can't get that information if parents speak for their kids. When given a chance, even kids as young as preschoolers can provide most of the information any doctor needs to know when they are allowed to talk for themselves.

>> **Don't overcompensate.** When a parent immediately apologizes about a future blood draw or promises a 1,000-piece LEGO set in exchange for a blood pressure measurement, that's overcompensation. These behaviors and promises may seem protective, but overcompensation interferes with a child's development of self-reliance and creates avoidance behaviors. Kids can do hard things and are stronger than you think. Letting them navigate nervous feelings with your support and guidance is part of raising emotionally healthy adults.

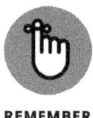

REMEMBER

>> **Don't forget we are on the same team.** Pediatricians have dedicated their adult lives to becoming child health experts. We are trained to put our patients' health and wellness first, while fully supporting the entire family unit. We want all of our kids to grow into healthy, emotionally mature young adults — and we know you do, too! Our advice and recommendations are meant to support this mutual goal.

>> **Don't ignore pain management.** Medical procedures can be painful. When needed, effective pain management techniques should be offered to every child. Supportive holding techniques, numbing creams, and distraction aids are evidence-based ways to reduce pain during medical procedures. Ask your doctor what pain reduction technique can be used to support your child through any necessary interventions. For more pain management tips see Chapter 18.

Chapter **8**

Walking Through the Psychological Evaluation

The psychological evaluation is an evidence-based, organized process that results in a child's mental health diagnosis. During the evaluation, experienced clinicians put together elements of brain science, child development, personal history, observation, and family dynamics to better understand how your child's brain works. After the evaluation is complete, you'll have the beginning of a treatment plan, including practical guidance to help your child's symptoms improve and your family move forward.

In this chapter, you discover the process of diagnosing anxiety disorders in kids and get tips to prepare for the assessment. You get the framework of mental health visits and the commonly used screening tools. I help you prepare for difficult questions, explaining their importance in the evaluation. Finally, I explain other diagnoses that may come up instead of anxiety.

Getting Ready for a Mental Health Assessment

Getting evaluated for anxiety is like building a jigsaw puzzle. It takes time to get all the pieces organized and categorized. Some parts of the puzzle are easy to see and come together quickly. Other pieces are hard to find, and some don't seem to fit. But by the end of the process, a clear picture appears. It's time to open up the box.

Selecting a mental health clinician

First, you have to find the corner pieces of the puzzle. These are the clinicians in your community who provide psychological evaluations. Your child's pediatrician may be all you need, since many providers will evaluate children for mental health issues. However, many pediatricians will not. Before waiting weeks for an appointment, be sure to ask whether anxiety is something your child's doctor commonly diagnoses and treats or whether they work in partnership with a mental health clinician.

REMEMBER

Anxiety lives in your child's brain and body. Your child deserves a comprehensive approach to ensure that the root cause and primary diagnosis is found. This process commonly requires more than one diagnostic visit and/or more than one clinician.

If your child's doctor prefers that you work with a mental health clinician for your child's assessment, they will have a list of recommended specialists. Often these lists include different types of clinicians with a variety of credentials and training. Find some distinguishing differences between types of clinicians who may be able to evaluate your child in Table 8-1.

The letters after a person's name are only part of their story. Use additional information from websites or personal references to ensure that the clinician has experience and passion for helping kids like yours. You're looking for a clinician with similar qualities to a great pediatrician as I describe in Chapter 7 and also confirming they have the availability and interest required to evaluate your child. And be sure to understand payment expectations.

TABLE 8-1

Common Credentials of Mental Health Clinicians for Children in the United States

Credentials	Title	Clinical Expertise*
PhD	Doctor of Philosophy	The highest academic degree in child psychology. Child psychologists can diagnose and provide therapy.
MD	Medical Doctor	Pediatric developmentalists, general pediatricians, family practice physicians, and psychiatrists can diagnose and also prescribe medications, if needed. Some MDs offer psychotherapy and counseling services.
PsyD	Doctor of Psychology	Child psychologist with extensive specialized clinical training in the diagnosis of child anxiety; may provide therapy.
PMHNP	Pediatric Mental Health Nurse Practitioner	Specialized nurse practitioner who can diagnose, offer psychotherapy and counseling services, and prescribe medications, if needed. Can work alone or with a mental health team.
LCPC	Licensed Clinical Professional Counselor	Master's level counselor with expertise in diagnosis, counseling, and therapy.
LCSW	Licensed Clinical Social Worker	Master's level social worker with expertise in diagnosis, counseling, and therapy.

* This list is not exhaustive. Each clinician's ability to care for and treat children may vary by state law, board certification, or licensure.

REMEMBER

Diagnosing and treating children for mental health issues is based on medical science, not personal beliefs or philosophy. Although there is room for individual style, you're looking for someone with a foundational understanding of mainstream medical knowledge. Proper credentials and licensure support this type of education.

TIP

Some mental health clinicians only offer assessments, but others offer both assessments and therapy. Be sure you understand what options are offered by the clinician you choose.

Preparing for the visit

Next, you need to organize and sort the puzzle pieces by gathering some of the assessment elements in advance of your child's appointment. This work will make your visit more efficient and productive. Many of the preparation steps from Chapter 7 apply to the psychological evaluation. Be sure to remember the following:

>> Clarify the purpose of the visit and what information will come from it. In turn, understand the number of visits expected with the clinician to develop an assessment.

>> Gather feedback, emails, grade cards, and comments from teachers, coaches, and other care providers to add details to the scope and depth of the challenges.

>> Complete any recommended surveys and questionnaires before the appointment, if the clinician requests.

REMEMBER

The diagnostic evaluation is a story. The story begins with your child's early years, continues with details of how they have grown and what behaviors you've observed along the way, and concludes with current concerns.

Explaining the visit to your child

This process isn't possible without your child! They are the border of the puzzle that holds all of this together. Gently preparing them to participate in the evaluation will make it easier for them to offer their valuable opinions and insight.

For most kids, it's important to give them a bit of time to anticipate and understand their upcoming appointment. Based on what you know of your child, choose an appropriate time in advance to let them know you've scheduled an assessment. Make sure to explain how the visit is a way to understand how and why their feelings and/or behavior have changed.

Young children think in fairly concrete terms and are focused on things related to themselves. Use simple and matter-of-fact language. Explain that the appointment doesn't mean anything is wrong, and they aren't sick. You may say something like the following:

>> "Just like we see a doctor for our body, this doctor helps with feelings. They'll play games, talk, and help us understand how to make worries feel smaller."

>> "The person we're going to see loves talking to kids and learning what makes them happy, worried, or even frustrated. There are no right or wrong answers — just a chance for you to share your thoughts and for us to learn how to help you feel your best."

Kids in middle childhood may be concerned about whether they're normal and the same as their friends. For these kids, the visit to the clinician may start like this:

>> "Just like a coach helps you get better at sports or a teacher helps with school, this person helps with handling worries or stress. They can teach you ways to feel more confident and in control when things feel tough."

>> "We've noticed that sometimes worries make things harder for you, and we want to make sure you have all the tools you need to feel better. This is just a safe space to talk, and you don't have to say anything you don't want to."

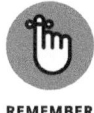

REMEMBER

As always, be truthful and direct. Let your child know that you're happy to answer any questions about the appointment, and explain what they can expect. Most importantly, talk about the process with a positive attitude and supportive demeanor. This will instill calm and confidence in your child.

Understanding What a Mental Health Visit Looks Like

The pieces are sorted and the border is complete. Now, it's time to start putting sections of the puzzle together. Through the process, the clinician will distinguish anxiety from developmentally appropriate worries, fears, and responses to stressors, while looking for other conditions that may be causing anxiety-like symptoms.

A comprehensive evaluation includes several parts. The following elements of the visit may change based on context, location, and familiarity with your family.

Structured interview

Diagnosing an anxiety disorder is primarily based on clinical interviews between the clinician, you, and your child. The interview differs based on your child's developmental stage, with more reliance on parent observation of behavior in younger kids and more self-reporting for older kids.

Elements of the structured interview include the following:

» Your child's story, including past issues and current challenges

» Family history

» Prenatal and birth history

» Developmental milestones

» Information about siblings, friends, and school

» Academic experience, including IEPs (Individualized Education Programs) or 504s

» Habits, routines, and changes at home

» Sleep history

» Nutrition and eating habits

» Behavioral observations

While with your child, a trained clinician uses art, music, photos, play therapy, or storytelling to understand your child's perspective, while watching how they behave in both structured and unstructured settings. This time spent together allows for direct observations of your child's activity level, social skills, frustration tolerance, problem-solving, and mental flexibility.

REMEMBER

During the psychological evaluation, the confidentiality rules in Chapter 7 still apply.

Standardized rating scales

Evidence-supported rating scales and surveys are tools that clinicians can use to support a diagnosis and monitor treatment progress. Most rating scales result in a self-reported "score" for the symptoms your child is experiencing. The score itself is not used to make a diagnosis. Rather, these tools are used to understand the severity of your child's symptoms at treatment onset and to monitor symptom improvement.

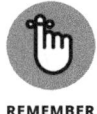

REMEMBER

Self-reporting is imperfect since it's hard to "put a number" on emotions and feelings — the severity of personal experience is subjective. For example, a score of 12 on a screening tool for one child may be associated with significant school or social impairment. For another, a score of 12 may be a comfortable symptom baseline.

Table 8-2 features a few of the screening tools you may see during an initial evaluation with a clinician. I introduce these as examples of the type of information you and your child may be asked, with the understanding that the scoring and evaluation of the responses requires context, professional training, and expertise. These tools are freely available online.

TABLE 8-2   **Commonly Used Mental Health Screening Tools in Children**

Screening Tool	Recommended Age for Use	Clinical Purpose
Preschool Anxiety Scale (PAS)	Age 2.5– 6.5 years	Parent reporting tool to identify signs of anxiety in young children. Assesses various domains, similar to SCAS.
Pediatric Symptom Checklist (PSC)/ (PSC-17)	4 years+/ 11 years+	Screens for behavioral and emotional problems, both parent and youth reporting.
Spence Children's Anxiety Scale (SCAS)	8 years+	Designed to identify the presence and severity of anxiety symptoms across different domains. Both child and parent reporting separate versions.

(continued)

TABLE 8-2 *(continued)*

Screening Tool	Recommended Age for Use	Clinical Purpose
Screen for Child Anxiety RElated Disorders (SCARED)	8 years+	Given in two parts, one is completed by the child and one by the parent. The results are given a numeric score that indicates anxiety type and severity.
Generalized Anxiety Disorder-7 (GAD-7)	11+ years	Self-report questionnaire for the severity of GAD.
Vanderbilt ADHD rating scales	6–12 years	Screening for symptoms of inattentive and hyperactive ADHD, as well as other conditions like anxiety, depression, conduct disorder, and ODD (oppositional defiant disorder). Parent and teacher versions are used together and both need to be completed for full insight.
Patient Health Questionnaire-9 (PHQ-9)	12+ years	Screens for depressive disorders.
BEARS sleep screening	2–12 years	Five-item assessment to screen for sleep disorders.
Children's Sleep Habit Questionnaire (CSHQ)	4–10 years	Assessment of behaviors associated with sleep difficulties.
Ask Suicide-screening Questions (ASQ)	10+ years	Set of four screening questions to identify children at risk of suicide.

REMEMBER

Screening tools can reveal symptoms you are unaware of, making you think, "Were there clues I didn't see?" But don't beat yourself up. When a child has an internalizing disorder, it's impossible for you to see what's happening inside their brain and body. These tools allow your child to reveal some of the unobservable symptoms they may be experiencing, allowing you to dig deeper into the type of support and therapy they may need.

Cognitive and academic testing

Anxiety can affect learning, memory, or attention — even mimicking learning disorders or ADHD, as I discuss later in this chapter. If one of these conditions is suspected, clinicians can perform developmentally appropriate tests to assess cognitive abilities and executive functioning.

Feedback and recommendations

At the end of a psychological evaluation, your child will often receive an *initial diagnostic impression.* The diagnostic impression is what is used to begin developing your child's treatment plan and obtain school support, like an IEP or 504 (for details see Chapter 14).

The following explains the important distinctions between an initial diagnostic impression and a confirmed diagnosis:

>> Impressions are made from early information and may change as more data is gathered, as treatment response is assessed, or as a child's brain changes as they grow.

>> Symptoms may suggest a few different diagnostic alternatives that need to be ruled out with more time, information, or treatment response.

>> Without an available brain or blood test (yet) to prove a mental health condition, an absolute diagnosis is not possible.

Anxiety is a master mimicker — it can look like lots of different issues (see Chapter 6). Your clinician's job is to piece everything together, not just focus on a few challenging behaviors. A thorough evaluation, patience, and time are needed to identify primary mental health concerns.

Expecting Difficult Questions

Some areas of the puzzle your clinician is trying to build include your child's personal experience with traumatic events and environmental conditions that affect the stability of your family. Sometimes, these inquiries can seem personal or intrusive. The following sections explain the reasoning for this part of the assessment, so you can better understand the importance of this discussion.

Social determinants of health

Social determinants of health (SDOH) are nonmedical factors that shape health outcomes. They include the conditions in which people are born, grow, live, work, and age. SDOH reflect *your child's environment.*

SDOH contribute to increased anxiety risk. Factors such as food insecurity, family instability, bullying, frequent moves, academic pressure, inadequate support, limited healthcare access, pollution, racism, crime, and unsafe neighborhoods directly impact mental well-being. By properly identifying SDOH, clinicians are able to connect families to existing community health resources and services for support.

Adverse childhood experiences

There is a close interplay between SDOH and ACEs, or *adverse childhood experiences.*

SDOH examine environmental and social factors that influence a person's health; ACEs measure an individual's exposure to trauma and how it is associated with personal health outcomes. ACEs are about *your child.*

ACEs are events or experiences that cause long-term or extreme stress. These are events that cause kids to feel terrified, helpless, at risk of danger, or physically hurt. The following list includes examples of ACEs:

>> Being a child of divorce

>> Being in a natural disaster

>> Having a parent with an untreated mental illness or addiction issue

>> Being in a school shooting or serious car accident

>> Experiencing a parent or sibling death

>> Being a victim of physical, sexual, or verbal abuse

>> Experiencing emotional or physical neglect

>> Having food insecurity at home

ACEs are not uncommon. World Mental Health Surveys estimate that two in five individuals have faced at least one form of childhood adversity.

ACEs and SDOH impact child development and long-term health by overwhelming their stress response systems, increasing the wear and tear of chronic stress during sensitive developmental periods. When stress becomes chronic, the physical body begins to suffer.

Chronic stress disrupts brain development, impairs attachment, and hinders social, emotional, and cognitive growth. These effects can lead to poor adult relationships, mental illness, chronic diseases, substance use, lower socioeconomic status, and premature mortality.

Although ACE and SDOH scores correlate with health outcomes, they are not deterministic and cannot accurately predict an individual's risk for future problems.

Positive childhood experiences

Positive childhood experiences (PCEs) are protective against ACEs and SDOH, and they improve long-term mental, physical, and emotional health. PCEs include strong, supportive relationships with adults and positive role models. Safe school environments and local communities are also protective. Kids gain PCEs with opportunities for unstructured playtime, hobbies, and self-expression. All these things create a feeling of inclusion and being valued that are foundational for wellness, and they can be identified through your child's assessment.

One of the strongest protectors against the negative effects of SDOH and ACEs is a caring adult who understands and supports a child's mental health. If you're reading this book, you are that person. Trust in the power of your support and the importance of your love and care, no matter how imperfect or messy it may feel. By learning more and seeking answers, you're doing the right thing for your child.

Exploring Alternatives to an Anxiety Diagnosis

As any puzzle-builder knows, sometimes the pieces don't join together like you initially expect. The mental health assessment can have similar moments, when the pieces just don't seem to fit. That's when it's time to look for alternative solutions.

During the assessment, clinicians are searching for patterns of behavior that may suggest a variety of mental health conditions. Sometimes, it's discovered that anxiety is not the primary problem that needs to be supported. Additionally, an alternative diagnosis can co-exist with anxiety, referred to as a *co-morbid condition.* Identifying these features may make a successful treatment plan for a child more specialized or complex.

The following sections cover a few alternative primary diagnoses and co-morbid conditions that can appear in a child's mental health assessment.

Attention-deficit/hyperactivity disorder (ADHD)

Both anxiety and ADHD can disrupt a child's focus. Unlike anxiety, ADHD symptoms stem from a core deficit in attention regulation, not stress-related avoidance. Kids with ADHD show symptoms in all settings, even during fun activities. Anxiety symptoms vary by situation, allowing anxious kids to focus when their anxiety is low or the task is highly engaging. Socially, ADHD kids are often interruptive and struggle with social cues, but anxious kids are more likely to withdraw.

Depression

Anxiety and depression are internalizing disorders that share similar biochemical pathways in the brain, making it common for one individual to experience both. Kids with depression feel persistent sadness, lack of interest, and low energy, leading to social isolation. Although depressive symptoms are more common as kids approach puberty, depression has been identified in younger children.

Learning disabilities

Both anxiety and learning challenges can cause frustration, avoidance, and academic difficulties. Kids with specific learning difficulties may struggle to focus on tasks and avoid certain types (for example, reading or math) because they are genuinely hard to complete. This struggle can impact self-esteem and social connections and lead to behavioral outbursts. In addition, learning challenges can develop anxiety and a fear of failure.

Neurodiversity or autism spectrum disorder

Children with autism often experience anxiety, and both conditions can involve rigid thinking, avoidance, and repetitive behaviors. Kids with autism, however, have these symptoms due to differences in social communication and sensory processing. Anxiety-like symptoms present when they are triggered by overstimulation, unexpected transitions, or unmet expectations. Diagnosing autism requires clinical evaluation by individuals with specialized training.

Obsessive-compulsive disorder (OCD)

The worries and fears in children with OCD and anxiety can be irrational, intrusive, and extreme. However, kids with OCD engage in compulsive and repetitive behaviors in order to reduce their stress. After completing a compulsive behavior, the anxiety quickly returns. In turn, the child feels forced to perform certain ritualistic behaviors over and over to prevent a feared outcome or symptom return.

Oppositional defiant disorder (ODD)

Both ODD and anxiety involve task avoidance and emotional outbursts, but the trigger is clearer in ODD. Children with ODD display hostility toward authority figures across various settings, leading to defiance and irritability. Limits, requests, and rules set by adults trigger frustration, anger, and arguments beyond what's typical for their age. Reassuring a child with ODD often escalates their behavior rather than calming it.

Perfectionism

Perfectionism is not an anxiety disorder itself, but it can be a symptom of anxiety-related conditions. Kids with perfectionism set excessively high standards, feel distressed by mistakes, and base their self-worth on achievements. Healthy perfectionism can help kids reach lofty goals, but unhealthy perfectionism can lead to excessive stress, procrastination, avoidance, or meltdowns when things aren't "perfect."

Sensory processing issues

Kids with both anxiety and sensory processing issues dramatically respond to elements of their environment, including situation avoidance. However, kids with sensory processing issues shut down or tantrum because their brain misinterprets sensory experiences — such as loud noises, food textures, bright lights, or crowded spaces — rather than out of fear.

3

Treating
Child Anxiety

Build a comprehensive treatment plan after getting an anxiety disorder diagnosis. Examine elements of cognitive behavioral therapy and other types of treatment, including finding therapists, determining goals, and affording therapy. Reframe common therapy myths that create barriers to accessing treatment, and how these barriers can be overcome.

Discover key principles prescribers follow when starting children on anxiety medication, and dive into the details of specific medications. Clarify the purpose, effectiveness, and safety of these widely used treatments while also addressing common parental concerns.

Review the evidence supporting the use of supplements in anxious kids, including details on effectiveness and potential medication interactions. Consider supplements with the framework of "buyer beware," including things to look for in over-the-counter products.

IN THIS CHAPTER

» **Appreciating the importance of therapy**

» **Revealing how therapy works**

» **Debunking myths about therapy**

» **Connecting with and affording therapy**

» **Gaining familiarity with therapy types**

Chapter **9**

Exploring Child Therapy Options

C hild therapy isn't just lying on a couch and venting about problems. It's goal-oriented work to help strengthen the parts of the brain that kids need to regulate and control anxiety as they grow. Psychotherapy is an evidence-supported approach for improving mood disorders in struggling kids, and clarity about how it works is essential. In this chapter, I explain the importance of therapeutic work for anxious kids, including the benefits and risks. I give you a comprehensive look into what therapy is and isn't, how therapy works to change the brain, and the impact of therapy during formative years. Finally, I summarize the different types of therapies that are used with anxious kids.

Understanding the Importance of Therapy

Psychotherapy is one of the most effective tools we use to help kids manage anxiety as they grow. Therapy isn't about "fixing" your child — they aren't broken! Rather, it's an opportunity to learn skills to understand their own feelings, regain confidence, and build valuable resilience. As a bonus, therapy helps you understand what's going on in their mind and how to support them at home, leading to stronger relationships and better functioning families.

Therapy for anxious kids helps them change unhealthy and incorrect fear associations. Fear helps us survive by keeping us safe from harm. In most cases, when the threat is gone, fear fades. But with anxiety disorders, the fear sticks around, even when the danger has passed. In therapy, working through how to shift fear-based thought patterns is a skill they can use for life.

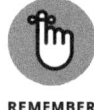

REMEMBER

Therapy during childhood acts as a prevention tool against future mood disorders. Unhealthy thought patterns become stronger over time, making child anxiety disorders a trigger for a chain reaction that can lead to other mood disorders later in life. Psychotherapy disrupts the progression of mood disorders and helps to strengthen healthy emotional expression.

Discovering How Child Therapy Works

The benefits of psychotherapy are well documented. Children who engage in therapy experience improved emotional regulation, greater confidence in facing fears, enhanced communication skills, improved behavior, boosted self-esteem, and better social and academic functioning. Age-specific therapy creates a foundation for lifelong emotional health.

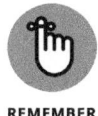

Broadly speaking, therapy works in three ways:

>> **Therapy helps kids learn about themselves.** The process focuses on learning how thoughts affect mood and behavior. In addition, it helps kids express emotion and correctly label their feelings. Throughout, therapy identifies the root causes of fear and worry, leading to long-term improvement.

>> **Therapy teaches and strengthens coping skills.** One of the greatest advantages of psychotherapy is its emphasis on skill-building and resilience. Through guided talk and play, kids learn skills they can use independently as they grow. These skills can reduce the risk of anxiety persisting in adolescence or adulthood.

>> **Therapy improves relationships.** Kids learn communication, empathy, and conflict-resolution skills. They better understand the impact and importance of their behavior on the lives of others, allowing them to interact more confidently and appropriately. Additionally, therapy can strengthen the parent-child relationship by fostering open communication about emotions and fears.

Psychotherapy teaches an anxious child how to reframe fear processing. This works by leveraging the brain's *neuroplasticity*, or ability to adapt and form new neuronal connections in response to experiences and learning. The various techniques induce changes in brain activity, specifically in the amygdala and prefrontal cortex, to strengthen top-down emotional regulation and fear memory association. In addition, stress hormones are reduced and neurotransmitters normalized. You can find out more about anxiety biology in Chapter 2.

To be clear, not all anxious kids need therapy, but for children who meet the symptom criteria for an anxiety disorder, therapy is often essential and highly effective. That said, even kids without a formal diagnosis can benefit from professional support, especially when facing acute stressors like bullying, divorce, grief, trauma, or suicidal thoughts. Therapy can also help young children develop healthy coping strategies and avoid disordered thinking patterns over time.

As kids grow, their first support is *you*. Validating and correctly labeling feelings, creating a supportive home environment, modeling coping skills, addressing and improving your own anxiety, choosing relational discipline strategies — all of these things are what anxious kids need. See Part 4 of this book for more insights.

Therapy for young children uses a modified approach and actively involves parents. Therapists teach feelings and coping strategies through play and storytelling, and parents learn how to support these strategies at home. This collaborative approach helps children build foundational skills, reduce anxiety symptoms, and strengthen their connection with their parents.

Reframing Therapy Myths

Unfortunately, most kids who need anxiety therapy don't get it. A 2020 survey in the United Kingdom reported that fewer than 40 percent of kids with mental health issues receive *any* professional support, and the data is similar in the United States. Anxious kids may miss out on therapy due to cost, limited access, or lack of awareness that support exists. Most concerning of all, stigma and misconceptions about mental health and therapy prevent many families from seeking help.

In my practice, I hear a few things about therapy that deserve reframing. Not only are these comments out-of-date and misdirected, but belief in them can directly interfere with a child getting the help they need. If you hear someone else repeating these therapy myths, speak up and correct them, or refer them to this book.

"Therapy didn't work for me, so it won't work for my kid."

It's not a secret that therapy doesn't work for everyone. Therapy is tough work. It takes the right therapist, at the right time, with the right environmental support to find success. As an adult, it's normal to feel frustrated and disheartened when therapy doesn't work out as planned.

However, your therapy is not your kid's therapy. Like every other medical discipline, psychiatry is evolving, researching, and refining its methods. Over the last few decades, great strides have been made in understanding childhood brain development and neurophysiology, as well as utilizing safe and effective methods to improve brain functioning. In turn, therapy has become more individualized and has an improved track record of success. If therapy is currently the most evidence-supported way to get your child feeling better, it's worth a try.

"Won't a pill work faster? Let's do that."

When your kid is struggling, you'll do anything to help them feel better. You want solutions now, and I hear that. I *feel* that.

REMEMBER

The choice to medicate a child cannot be taken lightly, and it's not the only thing that works. Medication can be useful to manage symptoms in the short term, but therapy is key to getting to the root of anxiety's cause, building resilience, and learning healthy coping skills your kid can use for years to come. You and your child's doctor share the goal of getting your child better as quickly as possible, and therapy needs to be a part of the plan.

"Can't I do this at home? I've been to therapy and know how it works."

You are one of the lucky few who have experienced the benefits of therapy. That puts you in one of the best positions to support your child's process. But you aren't your child's therapist. You are their parent — ready to offer love, understanding, and pride for the work they will do on their own. Connecting them with a therapist who can relate at an appropriate age level and use updated techniques is the way to go.

"They don't want to go to therapy, so we need something else."

It's normal for kids to resist things they don't like or don't know. For young kids, therapy can feel boring or pointless, or it can interfere with preferred activities. As kids grow, therapy can make them feel different from their peers or like they are being punished. For these reasons and more, it's normal for kids to resist therapy.

When kids resist therapy, it's important to determine why. When they tell you their reasons, acknowledge and validate their feelings. Find honest ways to address their concerns. Do your best to encourage them to continue or reach common ground on how long to try before they are allowed to stop. Talk with the therapist to see whether discontinuing therapy is safe.

WARNING

Therapy should never be stopped if your child is suicidal. In addition, if your child has significant symptoms that are disrupting their life (see Chapter 19), therapy should continue.

"Therapy is making kids weaker."

I've heard the popular media murmurings suggesting that therapy promotes "weakness" in today's kids. There are arguments claiming that therapy undermines parental influence, gives kids an excuse to avoid hard things, or promotes a pathological level of sensitivity. In my professional experience, this is simply not the case. For kids who are experiencing symptoms that keep them from enjoying the people and things they love, or kids who are navigating environmental stressors, therapy can be lifesaving.

REMEMBER

Therapy is not clearing a path for kids. In fact, it's quite the opposite. Individualized and child-centered therapy encourages facing fears, quieting harmful thoughts, and doing things that they would otherwise avoid. That's not work that promotes weakness; it's hard work that promotes resiliency and strength.

Finding a Therapist

In some areas, the challenge is not identifying a child with anxiety but finding a qualified therapist to help treat it. Waitlists to see a therapist can be exceptionally long, so patience is needed in the process. If you're interested in exploring therapeutic treatment, here are a few places to grab some names and start your search:

>> **Pediatrician:** Your child's pediatrician will have a selection of local therapists to explore, based on the issues at hand. Some pediatric offices have trained therapists as part of the staff.

>> **School:** Connecting with your child's school counselor or principal can help find leads. Often, they know local therapy providers who are near the school or providers who have after-school and weekend hours to accommodate student schedules.

>> **Religious center:** Your religious center may be able to provide faith-based options, or connect you with therapists of a similar religious background.

>> **Insurance company:** Insurance companies have lists of preferred providers, including Medicaid-approved therapists. Bringing this list of names to your child's healthcare provider can help narrow it down to people who are more well-known in the area.

>> **Personal recommendation:** Child anxiety and behavior challenges are common problems that affect millions of families. Asking a few close friends or relatives can often unearth a variety of recommendations to explore.

REMEMBER

If you feel like your child is showing signs of anxiety, start exploring therapy options early. You don't want your child to be in crisis as the search for a therapist begins. Treatment helps avoid the cascade of worsening and additional anxiety disorders, but give yourself time to find help.

Affording Therapy

Nearly all families bring up concerns about financial cost when I recommend therapy as an anxiety treatment option. The twist is that parents may feel embarrassed or judged if they suggest cost as a barrier, like they aren't willing to make changes or sacrifice for the well-being of their kid. Pediatricians know this isn't true — cost is a valid concern, and we try our best to help you find a partnership that is approachable and sustainable.

Depending on your area of the country, the following things can help make therapy more affordable:

>> **Health insurance:** Find out which child therapists your plan covers. Bring that list to your child's pediatrician to see who they may know or recommend from your in-network list.

>> **School-based resources:** Utilize free or low-cost counseling services that are provided by your child's school or school district. Asking the school principal is one way to get started.

>> **Community clinics:** Local mental health centers or community clinics offer sliding-scale fees based on your family's income.

>> **Nonprofit organizations:** Nonprofit groups that specialize in mental health support for children offer discounted options. See the Appendix for more information.

>> **University clinics:** Many universities with psychology or counseling programs offer low-cost therapy through supervised graduate student therapists.

>> **Payment plans:** Ask your therapist whether they provide payment plans to spread out the cost over time.

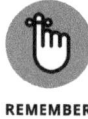

REMEMBER

Combining these options can help you access effective care while minimizing financial strain. If you need more help with affording therapy in your area, talk to your child's doctor and local mental health providers for options. The conversation can provide relief as you work toward your child's mental wellness.

Setting Expectations for Therapy

Therapeutic expectations specific to your child and family make the process more worthwhile. With a clear understanding of the structure of therapy, what a therapist can and cannot do, and your role in the process, therapy will be more successful and satisfying. Keep the following things in mind as you begin to engage:

» **Communicate commitment.** Just like anything else that is valuable, what you get out is what you put in. Let your child's therapist know that your family is willing to put in the work and receptive to any guidance they can provide. In addition, the therapist should communicate with your child about what is expected from them during and in between sessions.

» **Estimate the expected length of treatment.** Child therapy is goal-oriented. Being successfully discharged from therapy is one of the goals! After initial assessments, the therapist should be able to create a treatment plan that can estimate the length of expected treatment, based on your child's progress.

» **Define your goals.** Be clear and specific — keep in mind that this is your child's therapist and not yours. Goals should be focused on improving your child's healthy habits and behaviors, not "getting rid" of something or "fixing" your child.

TIP

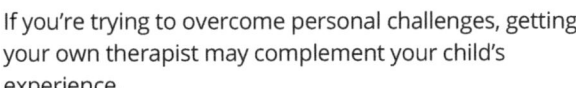

If you're trying to overcome personal challenges, getting your own therapist may complement your child's experience.

» **Allow transparency.** A child's feelings and behaviors are influenced by their environment, and successful therapy is tailored to a child's home life. If there is a significant issue at home, or one on the horizon, let your therapist know. This includes any medication changes, relationship issues, job changes, moving, or new family members on the way.

» **Describe your values.** Share your worldview with your therapist, including any cultural practices or religious beliefs. This will help your therapist create treatment plans that your family will prioritize.

>> **Expect highs and lows.** The therapy process isn't always linear. Stay flexible and curious. Identifying symptoms and patterns, and gaining insight to improve a child's functioning, requires time and deliberate, sustained effort.

>> **Know how your child's progress is shared with you.** Child therapy is considered short term, so progress from week to week should be communicated. Celebrate success along the way.

Seeing What a Therapy Session Looks Like

When families start therapy, they feel a variety of emotions including relief, hope, and uncertainty. Understanding what happens in therapy sessions can help demystify the process and set realistic expectations.

Mapping out the phases of therapy

Broadly speaking, therapy has three phases:

>> **Phase one is the warm-up.** The therapist focuses on building rapport, assessing your child's anxiety triggers, and setting treatment goals. Through conversations, activities, and games, the therapist will see how your child reacts to the process and determine their individual needs. By the end of this phase, the therapist will present a treatment plan and estimated timeline.

TIP

The more information you share about your family's goals and what successful therapy would look like for your child, the better the outcome. Clearly stating your goals while also understanding your role in the process, makes for the best working relationship.

>> **Phase two is the work.** It involves identifying avoidance behaviors and active skill-building. These visits may be with your child alone or with you, and include homework assignments to practice skills between sessions. This phase often includes safe and gradual exposures to fear-inducing situations, increasing your child's ability to manage varying levels of distress over time with guided support.

>> **Phase three is the follow-through.** This phase may involve occasional follow-up sessions to ensure that the child is maintaining their gains, or routine check-ins to refine specific skills. Once your child's goals are complete, the therapist will facilitate a smooth transition away from their support.

Child therapy has been developed with parents in mind. Family and parents are included in the sessions and involved in a variety of ways. Interestingly, the positive changes gained through therapy go both ways, meaning child-focused anxiety treatments also result in improvements in parental symptoms and family functioning.

Choosing online versus in-person

Since the pandemic, there has been a sharp increase in technology-based therapeutic intervention. Through apps and video calls, it's now easier than ever to connect with a therapist from your own home. These sessions are typically less expensive and more flexible to schedule, removing the barriers to cost and time that therapy often brings. In adults, internet-based therapy may be as effective as face to face. There is emerging data that kids can also benefit from online sessions.

Even though online therapy can work for kids, the strongest therapeutic connections happen in person. Just like the rest of us, kids get screen fatigue, are distracted by the family dog, and need to move around. Activities that build trust — like playing games, telling stories, or drawing — are more difficult online. Without strong self-motivation, virtual sessions can fall flat. Most of all, there's something powerful about eye contact and body language when connecting with a child. The subtlety of these connection points often gets diffused through a screen.

Telling Your Child about Therapy

The challenge with starting kids in therapy is that *they* are not signing up for the work — *you* are starting this treatment for them. Carefully introducing therapy increases the likelihood that they will participate and be successful.

When introducing therapy to young kids, it's important for them to know that they're not in trouble, sick, or being punished. A therapist is simply a coach, and it's always great to have a trained coach on your family's team. Keep it simple and honest. Compare the therapist to a helper they already know. Say something like the following:

>> "In two days, we are seeing a special doctor that helps us learn about feelings. They are going to ask you some questions, and me some questions, and then afterward we can get ice cream."

>> "There are doctors for our bodies, and doctors for our brains. Tomorrow, you are going to visit the brain doctor. I'll be with you during the visit, and I wonder what we will learn about how your brain works."

REMEMBER

Kids deserve the truth. Always. If a conversation is tough, share your discomfort. Share unease. Tell your kid you don't know all the answers. But when it comes to the big stuff — and mental health is big stuff — never, ever lie.

Choose a calm time to introduce the session, not in the middle of a fight or crisis. Often, it's helpful to talk about it a few days before the appointment. To introduce the idea, you may compare the therapist to a school counselor they know. Or describe how you've noticed they are feeling nervous, so you're going to a professional who knows how to help kids feel less worried. Let them ask questions in return.

TIP

Throughout your conversations about therapy, don't describe your child's behavior as a "problem" that needs to be fixed. Frame therapy in terms of *relationship*. Ultimately, that is what you are working toward.

Distinguishing Types of Anxiety Therapy for Kids

Several types of psychotherapy have been clinically tested and shown to help kids with anxiety disorders. Although the approaches may differ in delivery and specific skills, most evidence-supported therapies share the same core principles. The following sections introduce you to the types of therapy available in most communities.

TIP

This section is not meant to be a menu of options or all-inclusive but rather a tool to help you gain a broader understanding of the type of therapy your child's therapist may recommend. Ultimately, your child's therapist will determine the best treatment path for your child.

CBT

The therapeutic intervention with the strongest evidence of effectiveness in children is cognitive behavioral therapy (CBT). Due to CBT's success, entire books have been written about CBT technique, including several within the *For Dummies* series. For the past 30 years, repeated analysis and reviews consistently support that CBT reduces anxiety in children compared to those who don't receive any therapeutic treatment.

With the guidance of a trained counselor, CBT focuses on *cognitive restructuring,* or the modification of thinking patterns. It teaches things like relaxation, social skills, and gradual exposure to fears. Because it requires a certain level of cognitive development, CBT is usually for kids over age 6, though parent-child CBT can help children as young as 3.

TECHNICAL STUFF

Most children don't carry a "pure" anxiety disorder. Due to a child's unique neurodevelopment, most kids have a blend of the *anxiety triad* consisting of generalized anxiety disorder, social anxiety disorder, and separation anxiety disorder. CBT helps with all three of these conditions, not just the primary anxiety type.

CBT helps kids change how they think about and interact with the world around them, but this can't happen in isolation. Individual treatment is enhanced by family-directed interventions that strengthen problem-solving and anxiety-reducing skills. School-directed support also plays a key role by helping teachers understand and support a student's anxiety. For details about plans for anxiety management at school see Chapter 14.

TECHNICAL STUFF

Generally speaking, if there is no effect on a child's anxiety after 8–12 weeks of CBT, most clinicians will consider adding medical therapy to a child's treatment plan. International expert consensus is that the combination of CBT and medication is superior to each method of anxiety treatment alone, with higher rates of remission and durability. For more about anti-anxiety medications for kids see Chapter 10.

ACT

Acceptance and commitment therapy (ACT) is a contemporary method promoting long-term, goal-oriented behaviors rather than symptom reduction. Sessions focus on developing *psychological flexibility,* or the ability to accept experiences and tolerate negative thoughts rather than attempting to change or avoid them. Early studies have shown ACT to be as effective as traditional CBT.

DBT-C

Dialectical behavior therapy for children (DBT-C) is an effective treatment for child anxiety, especially for those with emotional dysregulation. The therapy uses well-established techniques that target emotional vulnerabilities and coping strategies. This therapy is modified for kids ages 6–13 years, and parent involvement is emphasized.

SPACE training

Developed by Dr. Eli Lebowitz, child psychologist and director of the Yale Child Study Center's Anxiety and Mood Disorders Program, SPACE training is a parent-centered intervention focused on reducing *accommodation behaviors,* or actions parents take to prevent a child's immediate anxiety or distress. (SPACE stands for Supportive Parenting for Anxious Childhood Emotions.) Accommodation behaviors unintentionally reinforce anxiety by preventing the child from learning how to face and manage their fears. SPACE training has been shown to be as effective as CBT and can be especially helpful when a child's direct participation in therapy is challenging.

PCIT

Parent-child interaction therapy (PCIT) is designed to help improve the parent-child relationship and address emotional challenges in kids ages 2–7 years. Through real-life coaching sessions, parents interact with their children while therapists guide them toward more positive interactions. PCIT helps parents have consistent, effective behavior management strategies while bonding with their child through positive reinforcement and play.

TIP

PCIT is particularly effective for separation anxiety.

Play therapy

During play therapy, a trained therapist uses toys, blocks, dolls, puppets, and drawings to help a child recognize, identify, and verbalize feelings. The therapist observes how the child plays, identifying patterns and themes to understand a child's problems. There is evidence that play therapy is helpful to reduce anxious symptoms, improve social abilities, and reduce aggression.

Therapies incorporating art, animals, or music actively engage children with passions in these areas, providing helpful additions to CBT-based treatments.

EMDR

During this treatment, an expert therapist combines eye movements with behavioral therapy. Eye Movement Desensitization and Reprocessing (EMDR) is primarily used in children who have anxiety symptoms that characterize post-traumatic stress disorder (PTSD). Children with PTSD have had their lives significantly changed due to events including natural disasters, school shootings, war, accidents, sexual assault, or serious illness. This therapy is rarely used for primary anxiety disorders in children but can be used in addition to CBT.

Preparing Yourself for After the Session

As a parent, you have a unique role during the therapeutic process. You aren't the primary therapist for your child, but your involvement plays a pivotal role in therapy success. Immediately after a session, it's tempting to pry and pester for details. Rather than asking about the session itself, let your child know you are available to listen and encourage them to talk.

On the ride home, keep the music low. Encourage your child to keep the electronics off and ride headphones free. Don't take calls on the ride home. Just *be.* Stillness encourages conversation. If they do share, validate their feelings and experience, and tell them you're proud of the work they are doing.

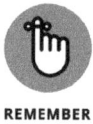

REMEMBER

Offer encouragement. Be patient. Commit consistently. Show unconditional love. Change will come in time. It must; that's what growing up is.

Chapter **10**

Anxiety Medications: What Parents Need to Know

For many families, the thought of giving their child mental health medication is scary. It's even more unsettling when myths and misinformation about these drugs remain so abundant. For families looking for medical support, I'm here to clear the air and help you decide if, how, and when medication should be part of your child's anxiety plan.

I understand medications will never be an option for some families. If your area has effective therapeutic, educational, and parental support for kids with anxiety, medication may be less of a need. This chapter is for parents interested in exploring anxiety medication as a treatment option and offers straightforward guidance on using it as a tool to help children.

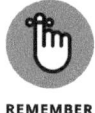

This chapter covers anti-anxiety medications, anxiolytics, and medications used for the treatment of anxiety. I refer to these medications collectively as "anxiety medications," the term used commonly by parents and pediatricians.

Considering Anxiety Medications for Kids

Medication is not, and should not be, the first thing that is discussed as part of your child's anxiety treatment plan. The preferred first-line treatment for childhood anxiety is effective therapy combined with home and school support, which is what most kids need. Anxiety medications are an additional tool used to treat severe or persisting symptoms.

Current evidence supports anxiety medication as a safe and effective tool for child anxiety treatment. Additionally, the combination of appropriate psychotherapy with anxiety medication has been shown to be the optimal way to reduce anxiety symptoms, improve remission rates, and potentially save lives.

A comprehensive anxiety medical plan includes three parts: therapy, environmental support, and (sometimes) medication. As you're exploring or debating your child's need for meds, don't delay inquiries into therapy options or hold back from making changes at home and school.

Understanding how medications work

Your child's anxiety is like a sensitive alarm system. When anxiety is uncontrolled, the smallest vibration of stress triggers all sirens to blare, starting a cascade of symptoms even when there is no real danger.

Anxiety medications "turn down" the volume of your child's alarm system. By balancing natural brain chemicals that regulate fear and mood, stressful triggers don't set off the alarms as quickly or loudly. That way, your child can use their anxiety-reducing skills during moments when they would normally feel overwhelmed. Once that happens, they are more able to jump back into the things they love and want to do.

TECHNICAL STUFF

The most common anxiety medication used in children increases the level of *serotonin*, a neurotransmitter involved in mood, emotions, and sleep. Additional details are later in this chapter.

REMEMBER

Child health providers would never want to *change* your child. Nothing is broken; there is nothing to fix. Having an anxious brain is part of who they are, and one of a million reasons why you love them. It's your support and care that will continue to help them grow into their best young adult selves — no medication can ever change that.

Knowing when medication is needed

Not all children need medications to reach anxiety remission. But if your child's anxiety isn't responsive to non-medical interventions, the choice to *not* medicate your child may further increase their risk of the long-term problems associated with untreated anxiety (see Chapter 4). Those are the complications that medications can help prevent.

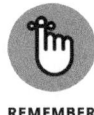

REMEMBER

Medication should be considered as part of your child's treatment plan when

>> Cognitive behavioral therapy (CBT) or similar therapy is offering no relief from anxiety symptoms after 8–12 weeks

>> CBT or similar therapy is not available in your area

>> Severe anxiety symptoms are impeding progress or limiting participation in therapy

>> A bridge of support is needed until therapy is available, especially in areas with longer waitlists

>> Your child cannot or is unwilling to participate in therapy

>> Your child is having extreme mental health symptoms, putting their safety at risk

>> Your child's pediatrician or healthcare provider may suggest their addition

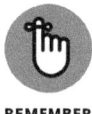

REMEMBER

Medicating a child for anxiety is a choice; so is not medicating a child. It's important to understand both the risks of *not* using medication as a treatment tool as well as the potential risks of the medication itself.

Finding a prescriber

Many pediatricians will prescribe anxiety medications, but many will not. As you begin considering medications for your child, ask whether your child's current doctor is able to prescribe. If they are not, ask where they recommend that you take your child for medical management.

WARNING

Certain supplements that I cover in Chapter 11 and commonly used medications may interfere with anxiety meds. Please let your prescriber know of all routine vitamins and medications you're offering your child.

Appreciating Principles in Medicine Management

Unlike fever reducers or antibiotics, longer-term medication treatment plans have different goals and guiding principles. In this section, I share a few guideposts that most prescribers use when starting mental health medications. In turn, I hope you will better understand a prescriber's perspective and your confidence in the process will increase.

Building a partnership

REMEMBER

Medical plans work best in collaboration, and prescribers depend on your help. A prescriber relies on you to observe and report changes in your child's behavior during treatment, watch for side effects, and monitor overall well-being. This feedback lets them make timely adjustments and ensure medication effectiveness. By working together, both you and the prescriber will create a supportive environment that maximizes the benefits of treatment and helps your child reach their goals.

Respecting individuality

Prescribers know all too well that not all medications work the same in every human. As a result, they use clues like your family history, symptom-reduction goals, age, side effects, and formulation — blended with clinical experience — to make the best decision for your child. However, it's not uncommon that more than one type of medication may need to be tried before finding a good fit, and prescribers anticipate the need for possible changes.

Targeting symptoms

Before starting anxiety medication, your prescriber needs a clear picture of the symptoms you'd like to see improve. Anxiety medications treat a variety of diagnoses and symptoms, but identifying specific targets helps track progress and distinguish side effects from expected changes. Most importantly, setting clear goals ensures better decision-making as the prescriber works with your child.

REMEMBER

Anxiety is a blend of genetic, environmental, temperament, and developmental systems. One medication isn't going to powerfully effect all of those realms. Narrowing the focus of what the medication is meant to improve increases the chance of success.

Recognizing that pills are not skills

Anxiety medications are not magic beans. As effective as they are, they won't erase symptoms overnight or make your child's life drastically different. Instead, they reduce symptoms enough for your child to engage in therapy, where real, lasting skills are built. Expect your prescriber to ask about your child's therapy progress.

To be clear, there is evidence that children can benefit from medication-only plans. If your child is in crisis, or therapy is not available or affordable in your area, medication-only treatment plans may be necessary. However, the point of taking medication is to help a young child strengthen the mental pathways involved in fear and worry. This is best accomplished using both therapy and medication.

Starting low and going slow

Anxiety medications are started at the lowest dose to minimize any uncomfortable side effects. Once your child's body and brain adjust to the medication, the dose is slowly increased until your child experiences symptom reduction. Although most anxiety medications work relatively quickly, it often takes weeks to achieve optimal symptom control.

TIP

Most kids expect medications to make them feel better fast, like when they have a cold or fever. Be sure to explain that these medications work more slowly in their body and brain so that they won't get as frustrated with the process.

Sticking to one change at a time

Therapeutic plans are built step by step. Too many changes at once makes it impossible to determine which change actually improved your child's symptoms. For example, if you started an anxiety medication, added a supplement, and started therapy all in the same week, it would be hard to know which part did or didn't help. Although it's not always practical or possible, expect your prescriber to make one change at a time to determine the effectiveness of each intervention.

Preparing for Your Child's Medical Plan

Certain details can help create a more effective medical plan for your child. Here are some things your prescriber may want to know to help them determine the best choice of medication or communicate progress.

Knowing your family history

As I explain in Chapter 3, anxiety is often a family affair — if a child has anxiety, a family member is likely to have been diagnosed and treated as well. In such cases, that person's experience with anxiety medications can guide your child's treatment plan.

Medications are metabolized by genetically influenced systems, so if a relative responded well to a specific medication, your child may have a similar response due to shared genetic traits.

Inquiring about insurance

Your prescriber will ultimately recommend and prescribe the best medication for your child. However, since many anxiety medications work similarly, the choice between agents can become a practical one. Insurance plans typically have a few medications that are "preferred" or less expensive. Knowing these options for your specific insurance plan can be exceptionally helpful to both you and your prescriber.

TIP

Tablets and capsules are often less expensive than liquid or chewable formulations. That's why the next section is important!

Practicing how to swallow a pill

Many anxiety medications are available as a liquid formulation, but liquids are more expensive and not commonly covered by insurance plans. Also, many of my patients tell me they taste "gross, disgusting, and terrible." So there's that.

Working toward the goal of pill swallowing can be beneficial as you're deciding on a medication. In addition, the pill-swallowing skill can be exceptionally helpful to stop the battles when your child needs any other icky-tasting medication, like a fever reducer or antibiotic.

TIP

In my practice, I see kids as young as 4 who are able to swallow pills, so give it a try. YouTube and other online sources have lots of teaching videos. How to swallow pills is also something most therapists will teach.

Defining your goals

All medical plans for kids need to be goal-driven. If there is no goal to reach, you won't know if the medication is doing its job. Before starting any medication, list the *specific* symptoms your child is experiencing. As treatment begins, refer to your list to monitor progress and share any relevant details routinely with your prescriber. See the later section "Looking toward your goals" for more details.

Prioritizing Safety

The final piece to preparing for a medical plan is to run a safety check. Hopefully, your child's therapist or pediatrician has already had a conversation with you regarding your responsibility for safety measures at home. If they have not, here's what you need to know.

WARNING

In this section, I talk very frankly about death by suicide in children. Please read this section with care and attention.

Straight talk: Suicide and kids

Suicide is a complex and intensely emotional issue. Suicide affects millions of families personally and deeply, and talking about this means of death can be scary and uncomfortable. For most of us, it's exceptionally challenging to apply logic and reason to something so devastating.

As a doctor who cares for kids at risk of suicide, and the families who love them, it's important for me to be honest and open about this topic. This includes talking about death by suicide directly and sharing what researchers have learned about how to prevent kids from dying by suicide.

REMEMBER

It has been repeatedly shown that talking about suicide does not increase an at-risk person's risk of attempting suicide. In fact, talking about suicide is one of the ways we correctly identify those at greatest risk and in need of help.

Understanding the risk

Death by suicide is rare in kids ages 4–11, but risk climbs as kids age. Mental health disorders, including depression, anxiety, and attention-deficit/hyperactivity disorder (ADHD), are prevalent in children who die by suicide. Additional risks include a history of personal trauma, neglect, or abuse; a personal history of suicidal behavior; and school-related, peer, or family conflicts.

It's well known that many suicide attempts occur during periods of short-term crisis, with little to no planning. For young kids, this most often occurs in their own home. During those fleeting moments, reducing or limiting access to lethal means of self-harm has been shown to decrease suicide rates.

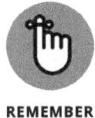

REMEMBER

Making your home a place with limited access to means of lethal harm is a vital part of a comprehensive suicide prevention strategy and a critical way to prevent child suicide deaths.

Reducing access to means

One of the most powerful and significant risk factors for suicide death is access to lethal weapons. For kids at risk, this means access to a parent's guns. The risk of youth suicide is lowest in homes without firearms. Among gun-owning families, the risk is less in homes in which all firearms are stored unloaded and locked.

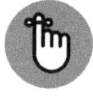

If your child is in crisis, the safest option is to store all firearms out of your home until the situation improves. For some families, this is not an option, or their collection is too large to move. In those cases, confirm that all firearms are unloaded and locked up and that the person at risk has no access to the key or combination. Use a gun safe, a quick-release safe, or a lock box. Store ammunition separately from the firearm, preferably outside of the home.

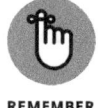

A suicide attempt using a firearm is more likely to be fatal than an attempt by other means. However, compared to adolescents and adults, young children who die by suicide are more likely to die by strangulation. Safely store common ropes and cords away from children, especially those that may be in their bedroom. Safely storing knives and other sharp tools is also generally recommended for homes with children.

Storing medications and other substances

Another means of suicide attempt is medication overdose. The following are ways to ensure that substances are properly stored in homes with children:

>> Keep all medications out of kids' reach.

>> Use child-resistant packaging.

>> Dispose of all unused, expired, or unwanted medications properly.

>> Lock bottles of abuse-prone medications in a medication safe, including prescription pain medications, muscle relaxants, antihistamines, acetaminophen, amphetamines, and mental health medications.

>> Keep small quantities of commonly used medications the family needs accessible, locking up the rest.

>> Store any alcoholic beverages and recreational substances away from children.

Maintaining bedroom safety

TIP

In children, the most common location in the home to attempt suicide is in their own bedroom. For children at risk, keep an "open door" policy, not allowing them to be isolated until the period of crisis resolves.

Completing safety planning

Safety planning is an evidence-based way to reduce suicide risk. A safety plan is a written document filled with personalized strategies a person can use if their thoughts of self-harm increase. Safety plans are individualized, culturally sensitive, and collaborative with a child's family and include specific instructions and strategies that can be used day or night.

A comprehensive safety plan includes

>> Warning signs or triggers of suicidal thoughts

>> Coping strategies

>> Social contacts or places that may distract from the crisis

>> Accountable friends and family who can offer support

>> Emergency contacts and professional support

>> Ways of making the environment safe from lethal means

TIP

All safety plans should include a contact number that is available at all times. In the United States, this is the 988 suicide and crisis lifeline. Find safety plan examples and instructions in the Appendix.

Again, death by suicide is rare in young children. The preceding sections aren't meant to alarm or scare you. Rather, the goal that I — and all pediatricians — share is for parents to be equipped with factual and meaningful information that will help keep children safe. Mental health issues are prevalent in communities all over the world, and understanding how we can take effective action to prevent tragedy has the power to save lives in all of our homes and communities.

Detailing Commonly Used Anxiety Medications

With preparation steps completed, it's time to deep-dive into the most commonly used medications for anxiety in children. This section outlines four medication families your prescriber may initially recommend, including those with the strongest evidence for treating anxiety in kids. Use this section to familiarize yourself with common options before discussing treatment and to refer to once a medication is prescribed.

Selective serotonin reuptake inhibitors (SSRIs)

SSRIs are what most prescribers initially recommend for the treatment of child anxiety. Interestingly, these medications were first used to treat depression, and it was only later that their benefits for other conditions were discovered.

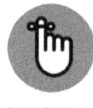

REMEMBER

Don't be confused by the *antidepressant* label! SSRIs have been extensively evaluated for their successful treatment of various types of child anxiety and have been used in clinical practice for decades.

Members of the SSRI family have names like Zoloft (sertraline), Prozac (fluoxetine), Celexa (citalopram), and Lexapro (escitalopram). The differences between the individual SSRI family members are subtle, with each having slightly unique neurotransmitter effects. On the whole, the actionable effect and medical benefit of each SSRI is the same.

How SSRIs work in the brain

SSRIs boost the natural level of serotonin in your brain and body. Serotonin is the neurotransmitter with an important role in feelings of well-being, as well as thinking, memory, sleep, digestion, and circulation. The benefit of SSRIs for anxious people is to quiet the over-reactive *amygdala*, the area of the brain central to fear and stress, allowing for more mental flexibility and reduction of anxiety and panic symptoms.

TECHNICAL
STUFF

SSRIs work at the molecular level by blocking the pre-synaptic reuptake of serotonin and enhancing serotonin-driven neurotransmission. Essentially, SSRIs block serotonin removal, making it more available to transmit messages.

Who is prescribed an SSRI

SSRIs are prescribed for kids with a variety of anxiety types, including generalized anxiety disorder (GAD), social anxiety disorder (SoAD), and separation anxiety disorder (SAD). For more on these anxiety disorders see Chapter 4.

REMEMBER

There is no "best" SSRI — they are all effective. Your prescriber's choice of medication is largely determined by family history, experience, type of administration, and cost-effectiveness.

What to expect when starting SSRIs

SSRIs are well tolerated by most kids, especially when started at appropriately low doses. Generally speaking, most kids see some improvement in 2–4 weeks, with maximum effect in 8–12 weeks.

The side effects of SSRIs are mild and most are *transient*, subsiding within a few days to weeks of continuing the medication. A few side effects are *persistent*, or continue until the medication is stopped. The following list details the most common things to watch for:

>> **Gastrointestinal (GI) changes:** SSRIs can cause stomachaches, nausea, vomiting, diarrhea, or change in appetite. These GI effects aren't unexpected due to serotonin's strong effect on the *enteric nervous system* (see Chapter 6). Most of these GI changes are mild and transient, improving by 4–8 weeks of continued use. The consequence to these GI side effects may be weight gain or loss, so measuring your child's growth at follow-up visits is important.

If GI side effects are bothersome, give the medication with food or offer your child smaller meals throughout the day.

Also, daytime symptoms can be improved by flipping the timing of administration to the evening.

>> **Sleep changes:** SSRIs can cause both insomnia and fatigue. In young kids, SSRIs are slightly more likely to cause insomnia, which is why morning administration is typically recommended. However, if daytime fatigue or sleepiness is seen, taking the medicine at dinnertime can help fatigue improve.

SSRIs are associated with regression of nighttime dryness. If your child starts wetting the bed, change the timing of administration.

>> **Headaches:** SSRIs are known to cause transient head-aches. But there is also evidence of headaches *improving* after starting SSRI therapy, likely due to the strong interplay of anxiety and head pain. Knowing baseline frequency and intensity of headaches prior to starting medication is exceptionally helpful. For more on headache management see Chapter 6.

>> **Dizziness:** Feeling dizzy or lightheaded is a transient side effect, likely due to SSRIs' effect on blood pressure. Changing the dose or timing of administration may help, but if this feeling is severe or persistent, let your prescriber know.

>> **Sweating and dry mouth:** These persistent side effects can be seen after taking the medication for a few weeks. Simple management with antiperspirants and lozenges can be helpful. In my experience, these side effects are not significant enough for kids to want to stop the medication.

>> **Activation:** *Behavioral activation* is a known side effect of SSRIs, occurring in about 5 percent of kids. Activation is characterized by increased restlessness, agitation, impulsiv-ity, hyperactivity, and sometimes even aggression. These changes emerge early in treatment or after a dose increase, resolving when the dose is lowered or the medication is discontinued. It's important to note that kids who initially experience behavioral activation *can* continue to use these medications in lower doses, with smaller dose increases, or in extended-release forms.

Serotonin syndrome (SS) is a rare but serious transient side effect of SSRIs. The likelihood of SS increases when the dose of an SSRI is high and when a patient is also taking multiple drugs with serotonergic activity, so be sure to share all medications and supplements that your child routinely takes. The clinical features of SS include agitation, confusion, high heart rate, incoordination, fever, sweating, and diarrhea. As soon as any clinical symptoms or signs of SS are recognized, the medication must be immediately discontinued.

TIP

Side effects of anxiety medications can be hard to tease out, because many side effects can also be symptoms of anxiety itself. Listing the type and frequency of your child's physical symptoms prior to starting to any medication will help add clarity to any possible changes.

TIP

When effectively treated with an SSRI, kids may begin to show symptoms of another mental health issue. Be open through the medication process to the possible discovery of new or associated diagnoses that require your support and care.

CLARITY ON THE BLACK BOX WARNING

In 2004, the FDA placed a "black box warning" on antidepressants after short-term trials suggested an increase in suicide behaviors after initiation of these medications. Since that time, large population-based studies have failed to conclusively link antidepressant use to higher suicide risk. Instead, research supports that *untreated* mental health conditions pose a greater risk.

Current evidence shows that when SSRIs are appropriately prescribed and monitored, they *reduce* suicidal behaviors by alleviating the symptoms of various mental health conditions. Although the black box warning warrants brief discussion, it should not deter prescribers or parents from appropriate treatment. Always monitor children for side effects when starting any medication.

Serotonin-norepinephrine reuptake inhibitors (SNRIs)

As the name implies, SNRIs work on two primary neurotransmitter pathways: serotonin and norepinephrine. The SNRI family of medications includes drugs with names like Effexor (venlafaxine), Cymbalta (duloxetine), and Pristiq (desvenlafaxine). Although norepinephrine is commonly known to be a neurotransmitter that *increases* the stress response, low doses can improve mental flexibility, attention, and mood.

How SNRIs work in the brain

SNRIs increase the level of serotonin and norepinephrine in the brain and body, while slightly raising dopamine levels.

TECHNICAL STUFF

SNRIs block both serotonin and norepinephrine transporters, reducing the reuptake of the neurotransmitters by the presynaptic neuron. In addition, SNRIs weakly inhibit dopamine reuptake. SNRIs lead to increased serotonergic, noradrenergic, and dopaminergic neurotransmission in the amygdala and prefrontal cortex.

Who is prescribed an SNRI

In children, SNRIs have been shown to be effective for GAD and SoAD. SNRIs may also be helpful when a child's anxiety is associated with low energy or poor focus. SNRIs may be prescribed if a child is unable to tolerate two different SSRIs, if an SSRI is not effective, or if there's a strong family history of SNRIs being the most effective option.

What to expect when starting SNRIs

SNRIs are well tolerated by most kids, especially when starting at appropriately low doses. Generally speaking, most kids see improvement in 2–4 weeks, although some positive changes can be seen as early as 1 week after starting the medication. Maximum effect is reached in 8–12 weeks.

Because SNRIs are working on the serotonin system, all the possible side effects of SSRIs that I cover earlier in this chapter also apply to SNRIs.

SNRIs have additional side effects including the following:

>> **Increased blood pressure:** In otherwise heathy kids, this side effect is mild and rarely reason to stop taking the drug. During follow-up visits, your prescriber will monitor blood pressure to ensure safety.

>> **Increased cholesterol levels:** There is a modest increase in cholesterol levels in some patients taking SNRIs. The cause is likely due to various reasons, including weight gain. This effect is reversible when the medication is stopped. If high cholesterol runs in the family, your child may need closer monitoring.

Alpha-agonists

Alpha-agonist medications are moderately effective for anxiety symptoms. This family of medications includes Kapvay (clonidine) and Intuniv (guanfacine).

How alpha-agonists work in the brain

These medications target receptors in the central nervous system (CNS) to dampen the stress response, improving physical symptoms and reducing impulsivity. Alpha-agonists also have a role in strengthening the function of the prefrontal cortex.

TECHNICAL
STUFF

To help anxiety symptoms, these medications target areas of the brain with alpha-2 adrenergic receptors. The drugs modulate norepinephrine activity and reduce adrenergic tone, specifically in the prefrontal cortex and amygdala.

Who is prescribed an alpha-agonist

Alpha-agonists are rarely used in young kids as a primary anxiety medication. However, these medications can be helpful for kids who experience both anxiety and ADHD or tics. Additionally, they can be helpful in children whose anxiety symptoms include hyperactivity, rapid heart rate, irritability, emotional outbursts, or trouble sleeping.

What to expect when starting an alpha-agonist

Alpha-agonists are well tolerated with appropriate dosing. The benefits of alpha-agonists take a few weeks to be seen. These medications are typically taken in the evening, since they can cause drowsiness. Other mild, transient side effects include headaches and GI upset. While your child is on these medications, their blood pressure should be monitored.

TIP

Alpha-agonists are useful as a nonstimulant treatment of ADHD in children. If your child experiences both anxiety and ADHD, this family of medications can be a great option.

Antihistamines

Antihistamines (H1-blockers) are selectively used for kids with anxiety or panic. These medications are found over-the-counter, like Benadryl (diphenhydramine), or by prescription, like Atarax (hydroxyzine).

WARNING

H1-blockers do not target core anxiety mechanisms and should not be used long term. These medications can cause significant drowsiness and cognitive impairment. In high doses, H1-blockers can cause seizures, heart arrhythmias, and hallucinations. Keep these medications out of the reach of children.

How antihistamines work in the brain

Antihistamines block histamine receptors in the brain and body, increasing sleepiness and decreasing the reactivity of the CNS. Antihistamines also weakly block serotonin reuptake, slightly increasing serotonin levels while creating a sedative effect.

TECHNICAL STUFF

Diphenhydramine and hydroxyzine work by blocking the histamine (H1) receptor, making histamine less effective on the target cell.

Who is prescribed an antihistamine

Antihistamines can be used for immediate, short-term anxiety symptom relief — not longer-term symptom reduction. These drugs work quickly and can help a child with acute or situational anxiety, but their effect is transient. In addition, these medications may be helpful for anxiety-related insomnia.

WARNING

Although antihistamines are commonly found in sleep aids, controlled studies have reported mixed results in kids. Even when the medications help with sleep-onset, some kids will still wake in the middle of the night or have too much grogginess the following day.

What to expect when starting antihistamines

Antihistamines begin to work in about 30 minutes, with peak sedation in 1–2 hours. The medication effect lasts 4–6 hours. Side effects of antihistamines are relatively mild, including dry mouth, constipation, and headache. Expected side effects are fatigue and drowsiness.

An interesting side effect of antihistamines in children is *paradoxical excitation.* In about 5 percent of kids, antihistamines have unexpected opposite effects, including increased agitation, restlessness, irritability, and hyperactivity. This side effect stops when the medication is no longer active in the body. Paradoxical excitation is more common in younger than older children.

Practicing Successful Medication Habits

Once a prescriber chooses a medication to start with your child, it's time to take steps to ensure safe and routine administration at home. The following are some tips to get you started.

Prioritizing safe storage

Risk-reduction practices and general common sense suggest that all medications be stored out of the reach of young kids.

Safe storage includes keeping medications up on high shelves, out of kids' play spaces and bedrooms, and in child-resistant packaging.

TIP

I recommend using a medication lock box for all over-the-counter and prescription medications in your home. Medication lock boxes are relatively inexpensive for the peace of mind they provide. They are available at pharmacies, big box stores, and online.

REMEMBER

To be labeled "child-resistant," a package is given to groups of kids under the age of 5 for testing. The package is determined to be "child-resistant" if 80 percent of the kids cannot open the package in less than 10 minutes — yes, only 80 percent. Although these packages are one valuable tool to keep kids safe, using a series of barrier methods to limit medication access is the way to go.

Normalizing a routine

Routines, like those I cover in Chapter 16, create predictable expectations that decrease unease and uncertainly. Once a medication is prescribed, decide how and where it will fit into your child's daily routine, offering your child opportunities to add reasonable suggestions to the plan.

TIP

For ease, I recommend a child-resistant weekly pill box. These cheap and effective boxes can be filled with the medications and supplements your child needs for the week, eliminating the need for large quantities of medication to be unsafely stored. Plus, these boxes provide a physical reminder to help ensure that medication is not forgotten during a hectic morning or evening schedule.

Avoiding self-administration

Young kids don't have the ability to self-administer any medication. Best practice is to offer the medication at a routine time and observe your child taking it. Generally speaking, most children are not able to self-administer medication until after puberty.

Expecting frequent follow-up visits

Starting any longer-term medication is a partnership between you and your prescriber. Expect regular visits after starting any medication, with the frequency declining as remission begins. Routine follow-ups and "med-check visits" are used to monitor the forward progress of your child's comprehensive medical plan. In addition, these visits help prescribers watch for less obvious side effects, like weight or blood pressure changes.

Looking toward your goals

Every part of your child's anxiety treatment plan should be guided by clear goals, including changes in home and school, progress in therapy, and symptom relief through medication. Without goals, it's impossible to know if your child's plan is working.

Choose observable and measurable symptoms to monitor success. Keep a physical record or daily diary of observations. Ask your prescriber whether rating scales (see Chapter 8) may also be a helpful tool. Share progress with your prescriber or therapist.

TIP

One bad day doesn't mean the medication isn't working. While on medication, kids are living dynamic lives that should include good days and bad days, so it's normal to see some ups and downs. Watch for progress by considering weekly to monthly symptom trends, not day-by-day variability.

Addressing Common Questions and Concerns

One of the challenges in getting kids medical support is overcoming the myths and misinformation about mental health medications. It's never wrong to be cautious or skeptical, but it's just as important to get accurate information so kids get the help they need.

In this section, I address some of the common concerns and questions I hear in my pediatric office. Hopefully, my answers will overcome some of your initial misconceptions and help you gain the assurance you need to continue the conversation with your child's physician.

All prescribers expect lots of questions, so ask them — and keep asking — until you get the information you need. It's important that you are confident in the process and your prescriber.

TIP

"I don't want to turn my kid into a zombie."

Your prescriber doesn't want to turn your child into a zombie either — that would be terrible! A properly supported kid should still experience the ups and downs of life. If a child is medicated to the point of emotional numbness, they cannot do the work to get better, which defeats the purpose of treatment.

"I don't want medicine to change who they are."

Anxiety medications don't work this way. In fact, it's quite the opposite. Medication can loosen anxiety's grip, giving kids freedom to be fully themselves. Medications are a way to reduce the symptoms of anxiety that are keeping kids away from the things they love and want to do. The only change to your child is that their anxiety symptoms will be in remission.

Emotional regulation and anxiety control develop through time, experience, and therapy. Medication is a tool to support that process.

REMEMBER

"Don't kids become dependent on these medications?"

These medications do not create addictive dependency, because they do not create feelings of euphoria. Anxiety medications are meant to be a temporary tool, and an experienced prescriber will have a plan to safely start *and safely stop* your child's medication.

Anxiety medications will cause withdrawal symptoms if removed too quickly. Stopping them suddenly without prescriber guidance is not recommended.

"These medications never worked for me. Why will they work for my kid?"

Family history of medication success is relevant to a child's initial medication choice. But just like personal experience with therapy (see Chapter 9), this medication is being used on a person with a different set of environmental, genetic, and social conditions than you experienced as a child. This sets your kid up for a different experience with medication.

"I've heard these medications aren't FDA-approved for anxiety. Is it safe to use something 'off label'?"

It's no secret that many of the medications we use for child mental health are not approved by the Food and Drug Administration (FDA) for the purpose for which they are prescribed. However, not having an FDA indication does not mean a medication is unsafe or ineffective. All anxiety medications for kids have gone through rigorous clinical evaluations. From initial animal models to randomized-controlled trials, these medications have decades of research behind them.

Docs use off-label medications in medical practice all the time, especially in pediatrics. Treatment protocols are not contingent on a medication's FDA approval. Rather, medications are used based on long-standing, quality clinical evidence.

"My kid is so young; will they need this forever?"

The goal of medical management is to support your child at the level and for the length of time needed to gain self-regulation, emotional control, and remission of anxiety symptoms. After that is achieved, many kids are able to wean off the medication with or without continued therapy support.

In a growing brain with *plasticity,* or the ability to change, unchecked anxiety leads to the development of disjointed, unhealthy brain pathways that further engrain and promote anxious behaviors. Controlling anxiety during this part of a child's life can allow healthier pathways to be formed, benefiting the child for the rest of their adult life.

"What about long-term side effects?"

A criticism of mental health medication use is the lack of long-term studies. But I'd argue that the goal of anxiety medications is not long-term use. Goal-focused planning includes using a low-dose medication until goals are reached, with a plan to stop. Extensive clinical experience supports using medications to allow children the opportunity to grow, play, and learn to their best ability.

"What if the medications don't work?"

Anxiety medications will provide benefits to most children. If your child doesn't respond immediately, your prescriber may alter the dosage or try a different agent to see whether it's a better fit. Rarely do young children need complex medical management for a primary anxiety disorder. If they do, or if there are additional co-morbid conditions that need to be medically supported, leaning into the expertise of a psychiatrist or mental health medication expert can be very valuable.

Typically speaking, if your child doesn't reach remission after trying two different medications or medication classes, it's time to pursue specialty help.

"This dose is the same that their father is on. Isn't that too high?"

Unlike other pediatric medications, anxiety medication dosing is goal-driven, not weight- or aged-based. Young kids metabolize medications differently than adults, so it's not uncommon that a prescriber may need to push a medication to an adult dose or beyond to see effect. Higher doses of medication don't mean your child is "more unwell" or dosed too high; it simply means your child needs more chemical support to reach the desired hormone balance.

"What about lab work?"

Many parents inquire about lab work prior to starting medical therapy. Personally, I think doing basic lab work is reasonable to ensure that no medical mimickers (see Chapter 6) are lurking, or to determine whether any significant nutrient deficits (see Chapter 11) are present. However, there is no requirement to have any lab work completed prior to starting medication, and waiting for lab results should not impede initiation of medical therapy when needed.

TIP

In the past decade, the availability of pharmacogenetic testing has become more widely available. These tests compare your child's genes — from a sample of blood or saliva — to a known database in order to determine which medications may be best. This type of testing is still an emerging science, and its current benefits are limited. For the otherwise healthy young patient, expensive pharmacogenetic testing is not necessary or routinely recommended.

WARNING

Fee-for-service lab testing has increased in the past few years through online services and companies. Be careful consumers and shoppers. Question accuracy, value, and hidden fees when ordering tests outside of physician-recommended lab centers.

Chapter **11**

Evaluating Supplements and Nutraceuticals

Spend more than two seconds on an advertisement for a nutrient or supplement on your social media feed and the avalanche begins. Ad after ad, celebrities and paid influencers, parents like you, all claiming [insert product here] will give you quick and effective relief from the exact symptoms you've been worried about . . . or Googling. (Funny how that works.)

Trying a popular supplement seems harmless. It's normal for anyone to think, "I'm sure this celebrity really likes and recommends the product; otherwise, why would they represent the company? Anyway, if it doesn't work, it's no big deal. I just won't buy it again. But, if there's *any* benefit, I'd hate to miss out!"

Add to cart.

This real-life domino effect — from problem, to influencer or ad, to "perfect" solution — is the catalyst for the billion-dollar supplement industry. All of us are susceptible to its power. From a physician standpoint, I don't ask parents to avoid these products entirely because some kids truly need nutritional support. Instead, it's about evaluating supplements critically, and using them only with specific and appropriate goals in mind.

In this chapter, you discover the significant challenges that exist in the current supplement and nutraceutical industries. With these concepts in mind, I offer practical tips for starting with and buying these products. Finally, I briefly summarize relevant information about the supplements I most commonly hear about in my office, including any evidence-supported guidance for using these products in children with anxiety.

REMEMBER

To be clear, I'm not endorsing or encouraging every family to supplement their anxious child. The data supporting most supplements is only mildly convincing. However, I know there are many kids with restrictive food styles, cultural differences, and erratic eating habits that make reaching nutritional goals difficult. My intention for this chapter is to help you make safer and more effective choices if using supplements feels right for your family.

Navigating the Supplement Landscape

More than half of all adults in the United States use some form of complementary medical treatment, including nutritional supplements. Use of these products by people with mental health conditions is even higher. Additionally, it's estimated that a third of children routinely are given supplements by their parents. And if you personally use these products, it's more likely you will give them to your kid.

Distinguishing pharmaceuticals from supplements and nutraceuticals

Significant differences exist between doctor-prescribed medications and wellness products available without a prescription. The following sections shed light on a few of these important distinctions.

Pharmaceuticals

Pharmaceuticals are what most people simply refer to as "medicine." These products are developed and made with the intent to treat, cure, or prevent disease. Pharmaceuticals go through very strict testing in labs and clinical trials to ensure that they are safe and effective before being approved by government agencies like the Food and Drug Administration (FDA), European Medicines Agency (EMA), or Medicines and Healthcare products Regulatory Agency (MHRA).

Supplements

Nutritional supplements are intended to complement the normal diet, provide essential vitamins and minerals, and ensure proper intake in those people who may be deficient. Supplements aim to support general health and wellness by filling nutritional gaps, not to manage health conditions. In turn, supplements cannot claim to cure, prevent, or treat disease.

Supplement manufacturers don't have to prove a product's efficacy or safety prior to introducing it to the market. Internationally accepted manufacturing standards for supplements do exist, but each individual company's production and regulatory practices are often poorly defined and loosely monitored. Generally speaking, Canadian regulations are the most rigid, United States regulations are the most flexible, and other countries fall in between. This lack of consistent oversight results in inconsistent quality and ingredients, leading to varying results with individual products.

Unlike pharmaceutical companies, the supplement market isn't constrained by enforced marketing guidelines. In turn, the claims a supplement manufacturer may make in ads or on product packaging are often stretched and exaggerated. It's legal to advertise these products as providing benefit to the body, even if there is no evidence from any clinical trials. As a result, our shelves (and social media feeds) are flooded with supplements claiming to be "natural" and "safe," and there are no repercussions for any company or influencer if a product doesn't work as promised.

Nutraceuticals

Nutraceuticals are at the intersection of nutrition and pharmaceuticals and focus on the prevention of nutrient-related disease. They differ from supplements in their purpose and regulatory frameworks. Nutraceuticals are foods or food parts that contain bioactive compounds and are considered food enhancers. There is a possibility that nutraceutical research could drive new therapeutic alternatives for certain diseases. However, like supplements, the current challenge is their lack of regulation across the world.

TIP

In this chapter, I use the word "supplements" to refer to both nutritional supplements and nutraceuticals as a single category.

Using supplements with kids

Parents give their children supplements to ensure adequate nutrient intake, support growth and weight gain, protect against flu and infections, or cover perceived nutritional "gaps." Additionally, supplements are medically recommended for kids with compromised nutritional status due to restrictive diets, certain illnesses, or other risks. When medically recommended, these products can be very helpful in reaching nutritional goals. But due to the lack of regulation and aggressive marketing tactics, determining an individual product's value is exceptionally difficult.

Directly due to the lack of production oversight and unlimited marketing ability, the booming supplement industry is powerfully influential — and parents are prime targets. Supplement companies have expansive marketing budgets, with the ability to get their product on every screen you see and every commercial break you endure. When bombarded with algorithm-driven ads highlighting a product's benefits, it's easy to *feel* that giving your child a supplement is what "good parents" should do, or that it's essential for their health. They are called influencers for a reason.

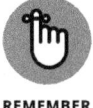

REMEMBER

Kids' bodies are smart. Outside of children with diagnosed food-related disorders or deficiencies, most kids will consume all the nutrients their bodies need through a balanced, healthy diet and don't need routine supplementation.

For children with certain medical conditions, physicians may recommend supplements to boost specific areas of the nutritional spectrum. Specifically, there is emerging evidence that certain supplements may decrease the symptoms of anxiety in children. However, in the current supplement market, ensuring quality and consistency is not easy for consumers and physicians alike.

Supplementing Smartly

REMEMBER

If you're considering supplements for your child, talk with your healthcare provider first. Nutritional guidance is an important part of any pediatrician's job. We want to help you make the best nutritional choices for your family and often have clinical experience that may adjust or add value to your supplement plan. In addition, we have access to various nutritional references and current research to help you optimize dosing, monitor for side effects, and predict success.

Starting with supplements

Any intervention for a child's symptoms — whether medicine, therapy, or supplement — should be tracked for its effectiveness. So, if you choose to start with any supplement, clearly define the symptoms you're trying to improve. Most supplements are recommended for short-term use (weeks to months).

If a supplement isn't reaching therapeutic goals within that time, it's time to stop.

Your doctor may recommend holding off on starting supplements if any lab evaluation is needed for your child's symptoms. Certain supplements are known to alter routine lab values, and these alterations may result in confusion about a child's primary diagnosis. If you've already started giving your child supplements, let your doctor know of any your child is taking, as well as any medications prescribed by other medical professionals.

High-dose supplementation should only be given under a health provider's guidance, especially for supplements requiring lab follow-up.

Understanding risks

Supplements can cause side effects. These can be minor issues like gastrointestinal distress or acne, or life-threatening contraindications like birth defects and increased cancer risk. Before starting any supplement, familiarize yourself with any known side effects.

Due to the lack of regulations, the quality and consistency from one bottle to the next may drastically vary. This variation can be especially noticeable when changing brands or opening a new bottle of product.

Supplements may decrease or amplify the effects of common medications. If your child routinely takes any of the following medications, be sure to ask your doctor whether your child's supplement should be continued or adjusted:

>> Antibiotics

>> Reflux medications, like proton pump inhibitors (PPIs)

>> Seizure medications

>> ADHD medications

>> Antihistamines

>> Oral steroids

Making better choices

As you are wandering down the supplement aisle, here are some tips to help you make better purchasing decisions:

>> **Read the label.** Choose products with limited fillers and limited ingredients. Things with sugar, dyes, sugar alcohols, citric acid, artificial flavors, and corn syrup can stay on the shelf. Simple is best.

WARNING

>> **Store safely.** More than 4,000 kids go to the emergency room every year due to supplement overdose. They look like candy, and the packaging isn't required to be child resistant. Keep out of reach.

>> **Consider the cost.** More expensive is not always better, but inexpensive supplements may have inferior ingredients. Compare prices on the shelf and try to hit the middle.

>> **Narrow the scope.** When possible, avoid complex nutrient blends or multivitamins. It's better to supplement with individual, goal-focused elements in order to determine effect. Some supplements are available by prescription. Ask your doctor whether this is an option.

>> **Look for NSF or USP certification.** The United States Pharmacopeia (USP) and National Sanitation Foundation (NSF) are independent organizations that develop standards to enable manufacturing companies to operate and produce medicines and food products of consistent, high-level quality. In turn, they carry out independent analysis on supplements and provide seals on those products that accurately reflect the contents. Keep in mind that although seals may help you determine what's in the bottle, they have no bearing on the benefit or risk to your health. Links to certification organizations are found in the Appendix.

>> **Watch for allergens.** In the United States, the sources of supplement ingredients are not required to be disclosed. This is important for people with allergies. Collagen, for example, can be obtained from seafood. Not listing this source can cause serious symptoms in a person with a seafood allergy.

WHAT ABOUT GUMMIES?

When shopping for supplements, it's impossible to ignore the vast array of squishy and sweet options: Gummies dominate the market. These products taste great, are child-friendly, and don't require the skill needed to swallow a capsule or pill. But are you actually getting what you expect?

Gummy supplements come with more issues than the common criticisms of artificial dyes and fillers. The manufacturing and regulatory processes also raise concern. The heating and cooling required during gummy production can break down nutrients, with continuing degradation as the finished product sits on the store shelf. To make up for this, manufacturers often spray extra nutrients or additives onto the surface of the gummy during the finishing process. This legal and intentional move helps the product meet label requirements after shelf-life loss, even if it results in a nutrient surplus at the start.

This leaves consumers in a tricky spot — you have no idea if your gummy supplements are fresh and potentially overloaded with nutrients, or old and lacking what the label promises.

Do these concerns make gummies harmful to your child? Aside from the usual risks of contaminants, cavities, and choking — no. To your wallet? Probably. If the benefit of supplements for otherwise healthy kids is minimal at baseline, the benefit may be even less in gummy form.

In my practice, I typically don't recommend gummy supplements. I prefer prescribing medical-grade liquid or pill forms when available. If those aren't an option or are too costly, I recommend over-the-counter pills, tablets, or liquids with clear lot numbers and expiration dates.

REMEMBER

Generally speaking, kids with a well-balanced diet will consume all the necessary building blocks for growth without supplementation.

Surveying Anxiety Supplements

Primary nutritional research in kids has grown throughout the decades, with a lot of insights taken from adult studies. Since kids' bodies work differently, some details about nutrition and supplements are still a bit of a mystery. To make things trickier, studies often use different methods and doses, so it's hard to know what really applies to all children.

Supplements should not be used as a replacement for or proxy to evidence-based treatment for children with anxiety.

Treatment studies for mental health interventions carry a high placebo effect, meaning just believing you're taking an effective medication can make you feel better. Anxiety interventions are reported to have placebo rates as high as 50 percent. Keep this in mind if you offer supplements to your child.

In the following sections, I note the strongest data for the use of a supplement in children when available. I also clearly indicate the popular supplements that don't currently carry evidence-supported recommendations. The supplements with the most evidence to support their use are omega-3 blends, vitamin D, magnesium, and iron.

Omega-3 blends

Omega-3 polyunsaturated fatty acids (PUFAs) are a family of essential nutrients. The two active compounds in most PUFA blends are eicosapentaenoic acid (EPA) and docosahexaenoic acid (DHA), and kids need both. PUFAs are found in salmon, avocado, plant-seed oil, walnuts, flaxseed, and dark leafy greens. Otherwise healthy kids are rarely deficient in fatty acids, but those with imbalanced nutrition or restrictive diets may benefit from supplementation.

In children, there is evidence supporting the use of EPA-dominant PUFA supplementation to reduce anxiety symptoms, as well as symptoms associated with ADHD and conduct problems. The effect of PUFAs is thought to be due to their influence in neurotransmitter systems, neuroplasticity, and inflammation. An acceptable dose for young children is generally thought to be between 1 and 2 grams per day, taken for at least three months, to determine any benefit. Ask your child's doctor what they recommend.

Vitamin D

Vitamin D is essential and is derived from sunshine and fatty fish. Vitamin D plays a role in bone health, immune system support, and mood regulation. There is some evidence that anxious people more commonly have low levels of Vitamin D, and there's emerging evidence to support supplementation for general mood improvement.

That being said, in otherwise healthy kids, vitamin D is one of the most commonly deficient micronutrients. For young children, the currently recommended intake is 600 international units (IU) daily. Supplementation amounts may be increased in children with confirmed deficiency.

Vitamin D is available in prescription-grade forms, which better guarantee product quality and consistent dosing. If you're considering supplementation, ask your pediatrician whether this is an option.

WARNING

Since vitamin D is fat soluble, overdose is possible and long-term use needs monitoring. Exceedingly high levels can cause problems with calcium levels or kidney function.

TIP

The American Academy of Pediatrics supports all babies being fed human milk as their primary nutrition to be given 400 IU of a vitamin D supplement daily.

TIP

If your family is vegetarian or vegan, it's recommended that your child be supplemented with essential nutrients. Based on your child's specific eating habits, recommended supplements may include vitamins B12 and D, iron, and zinc. Talk to your doctor to see what they recommend.

Magnesium

Magnesium is a nutrient found in dark, leafy greens, avocado, soybean, and banana. Magnesium is involved in almost all major metabolic and biochemical processes in the body, playing a key role in the functioning of the central nervous system. Stress, poor sleep, and strenuous exercise can result in magnesium loss or poor absorption.

Adult studies have supported the link between low levels of magnesium and increase in anxiety and depression behaviors. However, results are notably inconsistent. Stronger support for magnesium's use may be for bettering sleep, which may explain magnesium's positive effect on mood. For more on sleep and anxiety see Chapter 13.

Magnesium deficiency is rare in healthy kids; most get what they need in their diets. If you're considering a magnesium supplement, choose a form that is well absorbed, like magnesium glycinate, magnesium taurate, or magnesium l-threonate. Dosage amount varies by product, age, and weight. The most common side effect of magnesium supplementation is loose stool or diarrhea.

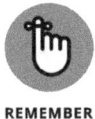

REMEMBER

Information about these supplements assumes that your child is otherwise healthy. If your child has a chronic medical condition or genetic diversity, speak to your pediatrician before offering any supplement or nutraceutical.

Iron

Red blood cells carry oxygen throughout your body, and they need iron to do their job. Foods containing iron include red meat, soy, beans, whole grains, and deep leafy greens. In a typical Western diet, kids are often unable to consume enough iron-containing foods to maintain desired levels during periods of rapid growth. In turn, iron is one of the most common nutrient deficiencies in otherwise healthy children.

Low iron levels can lead to *anemia,* or a low red blood cell count. Kids with anemia can develop a variety of health issues, including mental, social, and emotional dysfunction. For decades, it has been well known that kids with anemia need to be treated with iron supplements to improve red blood cell function. However, there's increasing evidence that kids with low *ferritin,* or iron storage units, can also benefit from iron supplementation.

A few studies have shown that iron supplementation in kids with low ferritin levels may improve anxiety symptoms, but the data isn't exceptionally robust. However, iron helps produce serotonin, dopamine, and norepinephrine, and increasing iron levels can reduce fatigue and irritability. Iron also supports better sleep, which may indirectly improve mental health. You can find out more about sleep supplements in Chapter 17.

TECHNICAL STUFF

Although international guidelines differ, screening for anemia is generally recommended for all toddlers and for children with significant risk factors for developing anemia. These factors include breastfed infants, premature babies, toddlers with excessive cow's milk intake, lead exposure, kids with malabsorptive diseases, and families with diets low in iron-containing foods.

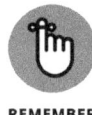

REMEMBER

If your child is anxious, exploring iron supplementation may be appropriate. Iron supplements are available in prescription-grade forms. Talk with your child's pediatrician to see whether this is an option and what iron dosing they recommend. For best absorption, take iron supplements with vitamin C. High-dose supplementation should be followed with periodic lab tests to avoid toxic levels.

Zinc

Zinc is a mineral that assists with various body functions, including wound healing, hormone production, and immune function. Zinc is found in foods such as kale, turnips, radishes, and watercress.

A link between zinc and mood disorders has been established. In children at risk for zinc deficiency, studies show that supplementation may offer mild improvement and potentially prevent anxious symptoms, suggesting a possible therapeutic role. In adults, zinc supplementation improves the effectiveness of anti-anxiety medication, but this mechanism is unknown.

Greater evidence for supplemental zinc exists for its use after diarrheal illnesses, providing immune support, improving growth delays, and during pregnancy.

Complex B vitamins

Low levels of B vitamins have been correlated with anxiety symptoms. The family of B vitamins is important in energy and neurotransmitter production, cell growth and repair, and immune function. Most kids get enough B vitamins in milk, cheese, meat, liver, egg, and green veggies. However, it's generally recommended that all kids on vegan and vegetarian diets receive a daily supplement of vitamin B12.

The effect of vitamin B12 on anxiety has been studied in children and suggests a positive effect. Studies on vitamin B6 are less strong in kids but still supportive. B-complex supplement dosages vary based on age and formulation. Most commonly available supplements contain a blend of B6 and B12, often with folate.

When exploring B-complex supplements, you'll notice high levels of vitamin B relative to the recommended daily intake. This is because your body absorbs only about 10 percent of what you consume. Since B vitamins are water-soluble, the excess amount is excreted in urine and not stored. Still, taking too much at once can lead to short-term side effects like headache, nausea, and vomiting.

Folate is a type of B vitamin. Although typically thought of as an important supplement during pregnancy, it's also reportedly beneficial for a variety of psychological conditions. Folate is included in most commercially available B vitamin blends.

Probiotics

Your gut is home to trillions of microorganisms, including bacteria, viruses, fungi, and more. These microbes happily live inside us, influencing a variety of physiological processes. When the microbiome gets less diversified, due to stress, antibiotics, food choices, or other factors, the gut imbalance is thought to influence various diseases and symptoms.

One popular way people try to support gut health is with probiotic blends. These products contain live bacteria (probiotics) and other compounds (prebiotics and synbiotics, which are combinations of prebiotics and probiotics) to nourish the gut microbiome. Although most people use them for digestion or immune support, there's growing interesting in *psychobiotics,* or probiotics that claim mental health benefits.

Research on the gut microbiome is still early, but scientists are starting to link gut health to brain health. Psychobiotics show potential benefits, but current evidence supporting their use remains limited. More research is needed to understand who may benefit, at what age, in what dose, and with what outcomes.

Probiotics should not be used by anyone with a weakened immune system or serious underlying condition.

Amino acids

Amino acids are the building blocks of proteins. Your body uses proteins to build muscles, repair tissues, and carry out many other important functions. Most of the amino acids are made by the body, but a few must be ingested. They are found in foods like meat, beans, and nuts. Without enough amino acids, your body can't make the proteins it needs to stay healthy.

Amino acids are used to produce various neurotransmitters, specifically L-theanine, a substance found in green tea. Tryptophan and tyrosine have been noted to be important for neurodevelopment. N-acetylcysteine (NAC) is an amino acid that plays a role in oxidative stress, neuroinflammation, and neurotransmitter regulation.

There has been growing evidence for the use of amino acid supplements in treating various psychiatric disorders, particularly autism spectrum disorder, repetitive body behaviors, obsessive-compulsive disorder, insomnia, and cannabis use disorder. However, further high-quality randomized controlled trials are needed to establish definitive guidelines for their use.

Lavender

Lavender is an aromatic plant associated with its calming scent. Typically used for stress reduction or sleep promotion, the therapeutic indications are based on tradition. In children, there is a lack of firm evidence that lavender flowers and lavender oil are beneficial for anxiety or sleep-related disorders.

WARNING

The use of strong fragrances in children's products or essential oil supplements is not recommended. Side effects have been seen with their consistent use, including skin irritation, respiratory issues, allergic reactions, estrogen-like hormonal effects, and ingestion risks. Never use oils to replace medical care.

Saffron

Saffron has been used in traditional medicine for centuries. Emerging evidence in adults suggests saffron may have mild neuropsychotropic effects and improve the symptoms of mood disorders. The mechanism of saffron's benefit is thought to involve activation of components that combat oxidative stress.

WARNING

Saffron is known to be dangerous during pregnancy, and high doses can be toxic. Until more is known, saffron is not recommended for kids.

Ashwagandha

Ashwagandha is a botanical that has been used in traditional Ayurvedic medicine for generations. It is considered an *adaptogen,* or a compound that helps a person resist or adapt to stress. Small, randomized adult trials using the extract of the plant have shown decreased levels of perceived stress, improved sleep, and improved energy levels with ashwagandha use.

WARNING

No systematic reviews support the use of ashwagandha in children. Be aware that this extract may interact with multiple medicines, disrupt hormone signaling, and cause problems during pregnancy. Side effects include stomach upset, nausea, and drowsiness, and the long-term effect is not known.

CBD

Cannabidiol (CBD) is a chemical derived from the *Cannabis* plant. CBD-containing products can be found on grocery store and gas station shelves, from lip balm to beverages and more.

CBD has recently gained widespread attention for its therapeutic potential in a variety of health conditions. Parents are turning to CBD to help their kids with ADHD, sleep, focus, and mood. However, there is not enough quality evidence to support the use of commercially available CBD to treat any adult or pediatric psychiatric disorder.

WARNING

Tetrahydrocannabinol (THC) is the psychoactive compound in cannabis that produces the "high" feeling. It's notable that independent testing has found detectable amounts of THC in commercially available CBD products. Although "isolate CBD" is an option, there is no way to be certain any commercial CBD product is THC-free.

Little is known about chronic CBD use or how CBD affects the developing brain. Potential drug interactions are unclear, and research findings are hard to generalize. However, CBD is an area worthy of more research, and more information and recommendations may be available in the future.

4

Parenting Your Anxious Child

Reflect on personal parenting behaviors and read about practices that both increase and decrease childhood anxiety. Introduce parental accommodation, one modifiable factor in the persistence of a child's anxiety behaviors.

Check out habits and choices that buffer anxiety's negative effects. Understand how protective factors, like movement, sleep, and healthy screen time, build resilience against anxiety as well as form long-term wellness habits. Appreciate the value of play, both unstructured and outdoor.

Look at ways to support a child with school anxiety and resistance, including when to get professional help. Help a child gain a healthy relationship with sports, and discover how to work through sports anxiety.

Explore effective behavior management techniques to use with an anxious child, including ways to discourage misbehavior and resistance. Examine how these techniques can be used while maintaining a safe and healthy relationship with your child.

Discover calming and co-regulation strategies, including the why and how of common calming techniques used with young children.

Understand ways to identify and support a child having a panic attack, how to get an anxious child to sleep in their own bed, and tips for successful co-parenting with an anxious child.

Chapter **12**

Analyzing Your Parenting Style and Anxiety's Impact

Your child's anxiety symptoms are influenced by a variety of factors. Many of these factors you can't control, like brain development, genetics, and temperament. However, external factors, like practicing positive parenting techniques, consistently modeling self-regulation skills, and prioritizing your own mental health are things you can control.

This chapter starts by reflecting on your parenting style and practices. Then you discover which parenting behaviors best support a child with anxiety. You also find out about accommodation behaviors, their consequences, and ways you can stop these anxiety-provoking habits.

Determining Your Parenting Style

Parenting a child with anxiety starts with *you*, as a parent and as a person. Analyzing your strengths and weaknesses takes honest self-reflection and can feel uncomfortable or expose vulnerability. I want to challenge you to embrace this potential discomfort for the sake of something greater — an opportunity to find ways to provide loving connection and meaningful support to your child struggling with anxiety.

One of the first things to consider is your parenting style. Parenting style reflects the overall approach you use to raise and guide your children. Style is a blend of emotional responsiveness, attitude toward parenting, and expectations for behavior and independence. It's shaped by deep-seated factors such as your own upbringing, cultural background, and core beliefs about child development. And your parenting style tends to be consistent across situations and time.

REMEMBER

Researchers categorize parenting styles into four main types, with each type influencing a child's emotional, social, and cognitive development in different ways.

>> **Permissive:** Permissive parents are warm and nurturing but set minimal expectations. They act more like friends than authority figures, imposing few rules while maintaining open communication. Their children have significant freedoms, like deciding on bedtime, homework, and screen time with little guidance or moderation. Although these kids often develop good self-esteem and social skills, they may also be impulsive and demanding, and struggle with self-regulation.

>> **Authoritarian:** The opposite of permissive parenting is the authoritarian style. Authoritarian parents enforce strict rules with little explanation and expect obedience without negotiation. They communicate one-way, set high expectations, and offer limited flexibility or nurturing. This style may provide a child a sense of security and encourage self-discipline. However, kids may also struggle with low self-esteem, aggression, indecisiveness, or shyness due to poor anger management and a lack of emotional guidance.

>> **Uninvolved:** Uninvolved parents meet basic needs but remain emotionally detached and disengaged. They set few expectations, provide minimal nurturing, and use little to no discipline. This style grants their children a high level of independence and freedom, often gaining resilience and more self-sufficiency. However, these skills are developed out of necessity. In turn, these kids may struggle with emotional regulation, coping skills, academics, and maintaining social relationships.

>> **Authoritative:** Authoritative parenting involves a nurturing relationship where parents set clear expectations and explain their reasoning. Children are encouraged to contribute to goal-setting, fostering open communication. This style promotes confidence, responsibility, self-regulation, and emotional management. Although it requires the most patience and effort of the common parenting styles, authoritative parenting generally leads to the healthiest child development.

REMEMBER

Each parenting style represents a distinct approach to raising children, although parents often blend characteristics from multiple categories. There is no "one-size-fits-all."

Putting Your Parenting Style into Action

Next comes another layer. Your parenting style sets the emotional tone, expectations, and approach. But it's your parenting *practices* that shape your child's development.

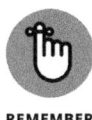

REMEMBER

Parenting practices are the daily actions — like discipline, routines, rules, communication, and support — that you use to connect with your kids. Unlike parenting style, which remains fairly constant, your parenting practices can change frequently based on new information, situational factors, trial and error, and specific challenges you face in daily life.

Parenting practices are also shaped by who you are as a person. For example, if you're a highly organized person, you may adopt more strict or structured routines, even though your style is more permissive. Or if you're highly extroverted, you may like to bring your kids to social activities and encourage social skill development, while being more authoritarian at home.

Successful parents adjust their practices based on the situation. For example, an authoritative parent may become more permissive when a child is ill, offering extra comfort and flexibility (for example, "Sure, you can have ice cream for lunch."). A permissive parent may become stricter when safety is at stake, enforcing firm rules (for example, "You're holding my hand to cross the street.").

This blend of parenting style and parenting practice creates the parent you are today, and the parent you'd like to become. The goal of examining your parenting behaviors is not to change who you are, but to be open to the experience of betterment over time. Parenting is meant to change and adapt.

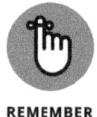
REMEMBER

You don't need to subscribe to just one type or style. Most parents use a variety of parenting approaches as their kids grow and change. Periodic, honest reflections of your parenting work is one way to improve the relationship and guidance your desire for your kids.

Linking Parenting Behaviors and Anxious Kids

Kids with anxiety live in homes with unique families and family structures that shape their anxiety experience. Research has specifically focused on parenting styles and practices and how they affect a child's anxiety symptoms, duration, and severity. After decades of work, some consistent themes have been revealed, as you find out in the following sections.

REMEMBER

Many factors contribute to the development of anxiety, like inhibited temperament, school and peer experiences, and biological development. You can find out more about predictors of child anxiety in Chapter 3.

Contributing to child anxiety

Parenting behaviors are critical environmental factors that influence the experience of child anxiety. Specifically, control-related parenting behaviors, like overprotection, excessive reassurance, and excessive guidance focus too strongly on the dangers of the outside world, leading to the development of child anxiety.

>> **Over-involved parenting behaviors limit a child's independence, reinforce fear, and hinder coping skill development.** Well-meaning "helicopter parents" intervene to prevent struggles, but these behaviors inadvertently teach kids that they can't handle certain challenges, emotions, or situations on their own. As a result, these children struggle with emotional regulation, have lower confidence in peer relationships, and develop heightened stress responses, increasing their risk of generalized and social anxiety.

>> **Excessive reassurance limits a child's engagement and reinforces avoidance.** I see parents try to "rescue" their kids nearly every day in my pediatric office, especially when kids feel (appropriately) nervous before exams or vaccinations. Parents mean well, but too much reassurance signals that the exam is, in fact, scary — making children withdraw and resist interacting with me.

>> **Constantly giving children specific instructions interferes with developing independence.** "Micromanaging moments" limit opportunities for choice and self-direction. When children have little control regarding their ability to independently manage their environments, they start to feel less confident and more anxious because they're not used to handling things independently.

>> **Overly critical parenting behaviors contribute to the development of pathological anxiety in children.** Harshness is one of the main characteristics of authoritarian parenting behaviors, as well as yelling, scolding, and shaming. Exposure to these types of verbal aggression makes kids fearful of mistakes and punishment. Additionally, constant criticism fosters self-doubt, making it hard for kids to express themselves or make decisions. As a result, they may feel isolated and uncertain, intensifying anxiety and lowering self-esteem.

Protecting against anxiety

Awareness of your personal tendencies and patterns is the first step in engaging with and supporting your child with anxiety. The following are parenting behaviors that decrease the likelihood of childhood anxiety and foster emotional resilience:

>> **Encouraging independence:** Allowing children to solve problems, make age-appropriate decisions, and experience manageable challenges fosters self-efficacy. This reduces anxiety by reinforcing a sense of competence.

>> **Setting clear expectations:** Studies show that parenting behaviors associated with the authoritative parenting style that warmly set clear and reproducible expectations help children develop secure attachment, emotional regulation, and resilience against anxiety.

>> **Allowing exposure to challenges:** Gradual exposure to feared situations strengthens coping mechanisms, fosters relationships, and reduces avoidance behaviors. During these moments, some gentle reassurance is helpful, without repeatedly assuring them that everything will be all right.

>> **Validating without catastrophizing:** Parental validation of emotions without reinforcing catastrophic thinking helps children develop emotional regulation rather than excessive fear.

>> **Being consistent but flexible:** Predictable routines and clear expectations provide children with a sense of security, reducing uncertainty-driven anxiety. Flexibility with routines can help kids adapt to new situations. Find out more in Chapter 13.

>> **Modeling coping skills:** Parents who model calm responses to stress, use positive reframing, and encourage problem-solving over avoidance help their children develop strong emotional regulation.

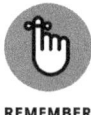

Anxiety is not always preventable, but there are ways to modify internal and external factors that can improve and shorten a child's experience with anxiety.

Reflecting on your parenting behaviors

Okay, let's be real for a minute. After reading the previous sections, did a parenting habit come to mind that may be *adding* to your child's anxiety? That's normal. We all have behaviors we're not proud of or feel stuck in. The goal of this reflection isn't to blame, shame, or justify — it's to recognize patterns, understand their impact, and consider a different approach when you're ready.

TIP

Just like you give your kids grace for mistakes, give grace to yourself. Parenting is not easy for anyone, no matter what their social media feed may imply. Honor your willingness to learn and adapt — not every parent is! Give yourself time and space to learn what's going to work best for your unique family.

Parenting with Anxiety

Routinely practicing parenting behaviors that support a child's social-emotional growth isn't easy. It takes patience, focus, time, and dedication that not every parent is capable of, despite the best of intentions. An additional factor also makes practicing anxiety-preventing parenting behaviors nearly impossible — when *you* have anxiety, too.

If you're reading this book, you probably have some experience with anxiety. In fact, I assume you do. Anxiety is one of the leading mental health disorders in adults, and for similar reasons to those I give in Chapter 3, anxiety is on the rise in adults worldwide. Also, anxiety is shared genetically. If a child has anxiety, there's about a 40 percent chance that at least one parent can relate to the irrational fears and worries that anxiety can cause. Is this you?

If you're struggling with anxiety, parenting feels more challenging, and it feels this way for good reason. Anxiety changes your parenting practices, creates barriers in your parent-child relationship, and alters your parenting experience in ways that you may or may not be aware of. The following sections explain what research suggests about how anxiety influences your parenting behaviors.

Anxiety intercepts your parenting effectiveness

Anxious parents often worry excessively about their child's well-being, becoming overly controlling or hesitant to set boundaries — traits of authoritarian or permissive styles. They may overprotect, detach emotionally, or set inconsistent expectations. Anxiety also weakens problem-solving, leading to inconsistent discipline, overreactions, and decision-making struggles. Over time, these patterns confuse children, strain the parent-child bond, and reduce parenting effectiveness.

Anxiety intensifies your child's experience with anxiety

Parents affected by anxiety disorders don't have the ability to co-regulate. All their energy is focused on controlling their own emotional response during stressful moments, with none to spare for their kids. Meanwhile, the parents' own maladaptive anxiety behaviors, like accommodation or avoidance, may be the only practice their child sees. Over time, children may mirror these anxious patterns, making the child feel less secure and develop a heightened stress response.

Anxiety makes your emotional interpretations inaccurate

Anxiety can interfere with a parent's ability to accurately identify your child's emotions. For example, say you and your child are visiting the zoo. During the visit, a zookeeper is safely holding and showing a spider to the group, but your child doesn't want to touch the spider. If you have a phobia of spiders, you may quickly grab them away, tell them it's okay to be scared, and encourage them to avoid the spider. In this moment, your anxiety prevents you from recognizing your child's fear as normal and age-appropriate, potentially increasing the risk of your child developing a phobia as they grow.

Anxiety is contagious

Kids look to parents for cues — both good and bad. They notice how you handle stress just as much as your table manners or how you greet the mail carrier. If you show anxious or fearful behaviors, those are modeled as well.

A child's mental health struggles can also directly impact a parent's well-being through emotional patterning, mutual distress, and increased caregiving demands. This two-way effect raises parental stress, burnout, and the risk of anxiety and depression.

Anxiety changes your parenting memories

Uncontrolled anxiety interferes with memory development by disrupting key brain functions involved in learning and recall. This makes it harder to encode and retrieve information effectively. Additionally, anxiety diverts your cognitive resources, forcing the brain to focus on perceived threats rather than absorbing new information. Over time, this constant state of worry can weaken your working memory, making it difficult to retain and process details, and to recall past experiences.

Anxiety interferes with your relationships

Anxiety makes people overly fearful, irritable, or withdrawn. As a parent, these disruptions make it harder for you to offer consistent warmth and reassurance. You may be less emotionally available while being more demanding, punitive, and harsh. This leads to over-reactive moments with your kids, impulsive and erratic discipline, and inconsistency that erodes trust.

Anxiety steals your parenting joy

Uncontrolled anxiety drains parental joy, increasing stress, exhaustion, and difficulty staying present. It makes it hard to relax and enjoy daily moments with your child. Anxious parents focus on dangers and mistakes instead of small wins and moments of connection. Additionally, studies show high anxiety lowers parental confidence, leading to frustration instead of fulfillment. Over time, constant worry turns parenting into a burden rather than a rewarding experience.

Anxiety is worth treating

A parent's anxiety deserves treatment not only for their own well-being but also for their child's emotional health and development. For you, untreated anxiety can lead to chronic stress, exhaustion, and difficulty managing daily responsibilities, making life feel overwhelming. For your child, anxious parenting can create an unpredictable environment, reinforcing fear, overprotection, or emotional withdrawal, all of which increase a child's risk of developing anxiety themselves.

By seeking treatment — whether through therapy, medication, or lifestyle changes — parents can model healthy coping strategies, regulate their own emotions, and create a calmer, more secure environment where their child can thrive.

REMEMBER

Your child's anxiety isn't your fault or a reflection of you as a parent. But supporting them starts with taking care of your own mental health. Sometimes, that means seeking help. Prioritizing your well-being is one of the most loving and impactful ways to support your child's long-term health and safety.

Avoiding Accommodation

Your main role as a parent of an anxious kid is to offer effective and consistent support, calm confidence, and love. But during anxious moments, it's never simple, never easy. As a result of the difficulty that consistent anxiety support requires, it's not uncommon that parents develop accommodation behaviors.

Accommodation behaviors are actions parents take to help their kids avoid an anxiety-provoking experience. Accommodation includes adhering to strict child-assigned "rules," modifying family routines, and providing excessive reassurance —

specifically to avoid their child getting stressed. These are not behaviors parents *want* to do. Rather, accommodations are things they feel they *have* to do to keep their child comfortable.

Common accommodations include small routine changes, like leaving a light on at night or making separate meals at dinner-time. Other accommodations start small but escalate, like answering obsessive questions or navigating lengthy bedtime routines.

WARNING

The longer accommodations are used, the more anxiety is increased by reinforcing fear, hindering coping skill develop-ment, and heightening the stress response.

Discovering your accommodation behaviors

So, how do you know whether you're accommodating? Ask yourself the following two questions:

❯❯ Is this behavior making my child more independent and ready to take on a next step or goal?

❯❯ Is this behavior making me resentful, unhappy, or interfer-ing with something else I'd rather be doing?

Accommodation behaviors directly interfere with the develop-ment of independence. So, if you answered "no" to question one, you may be accommodating. Additionally, accommodation behaviors get weary over time, disrupt family function, and ulti-mately interfere with your relationship with your child. That's a "yes" to question two.

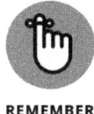

REMEMBER

Improving anxiety requires controlled and consistent exposure to things or situations that cause stress. Supporting your child through these moments is how you show love, understanding, and care. If you're accommodating, you're hindering the healing guidance that you have the power to provide. Plus, you're extending the duration and durability of your child's experience with anxiety, making it harder for them to move into remission.

Stopping accommodation

Consistent and proper support will teach your child that they have the competence to handle stressful situations. This will help you gain greater calm in your home over time. If you are accommodating and are ready to stop, the following are tips to gently approach this change:

» **Make a list of your accommodation behaviors.** You likely have more than one. Take note when you change a routine, provide excessive reassurance, or avoid situations to reduce your child's anxiety. Keep track of patterns.

» **Communicate the change.** Have an open conversation with your child about facing fears gradually. Use age-appropriate language to explain why avoidance won't help them grow.

» **Start small.** Pick one accommodation to reduce at a time. Pick something that happens often enough that you can work on it frequently and measure the results. For example, if your child asks for six stories at bedtime, read two stories.

» **Explain and rehearse the plan.** Explain the change you're going to make to your child. Practice the plan during times of calm, before the stressful moment arrives. Allow your child to ask questions or modify the plan if it seems to be a reasonable step toward the progress you desire, but don't leave room for arguments or negotiations.

» **Use supportive language.** Replace excessive reassurance with encouragement. Instead of "You'll be fine; don't worry," try "I know this is hard, but I believe you can handle it."

» **Reward effort, not just success.** Praise your child for trying, even if they struggle. Celebrate small wins to build confidence.

» **Know your limits and when you need to disengage.** If your child's reaction to the new plan is too overwhelming for you to handle, know when you need to change course. Alternatively, working with a therapist to create a structured plan can be empowering and necessary to reduce accommodations. Find links to helpful sources in the Appendix.

IN THIS CHAPTER

» Protecting against the negative
effects of stress

» Improving sleep for your anxious
child

» Moving and fueling the anxious
brain

» Navigating screen time, play, and
routines

Chapter **13**

Optimizing Your Home Environment

elcome to the most important chapter in this book. These pages remove all the things about your anxious child that you can't control, and focus your efforts on the things you can. Some of these things may surprise you — a few may astound you. All of them promote and encourage your entire family's mental health.

In this chapter, you discover why supporting an anxious child begins at home. I describe ways sleep, exercise, and nutrition form the building blocks of mental wellness. You gain practical tips to prioritize healthy goals, including play and screen time. You find out how placing these goals within predictable structure decreases your child's anxiety. Along the way, I encourage you to take small, meaningful steps forward.

Understanding That Anxiety Management Starts at Home

At first glance, you may be tempted to skip over what most parents already know to be healthy habits, like eating nutritious food, getting great sleep, and exercising routinely. But effectively managing your home environment helps your kids have a healthier relationship with their given genetics and innate temperament. These are not just "good ideas," but intentional steps to protect mental wellness.

Stress and anxiety are an inevitable part of life, so it's crucial to proactively construct defenses to shield your family from their impact. Sleep, nutrition, movement, and more — all of these things protect against anxiety's negative effects. You have the power to shape these things for your family. Kids can't do this on their own.

The commitment to creating protective defenses against anxiety requires parental leadership, which can feel exceptionally hard, so please don't get overwhelmed. Rather, prioritize one of these powerful resilience factors at a time. Every choice you make will create a positive change that benefits your anxious child and whole family.

REMEMBER

Parenting is a high-stakes job, and there's no one better to do it for your child than you. Not every day is perfect, and there are exceptions to every rule, but making the choice to prioritize sleep, nutrition, exercise, screens, play, and routines will never be a decision you regret.

Prioritizing Sleep

Sleep is essential for our physical and mental health, yet it's exceptionally complex. Sleep is personal, culturally driven, and unique to every family. In addition, each child has distinctive neurodevelopment, temperament, and internal health conditions that also affect sleep. These variables and more make it difficult to define "good sleep" or offer generalized sleep guidance.

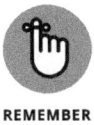

Despite innate challenges in the field of sleep science, we still find valuable insight when looking at existing research as a whole. By combining primary sleep research with more generalized conclusions, consistent, reproducible themes for better sleep percolate to the top:

>> Sleep is vital for your child's health, and poor sleep is strongly connected with mental, emotional, and physical problems.

>> Kids' sleep quality directly affects family function and parental mental health.

>> Kids with anxiety commonly have sleep challenges, often directly related to the biologic changes in the anxious brain.

>> From infancy through the teenage years, kids depend on parents and caregivers to make great sleep happen.

>> Sleep quality and quantity can be improved.

Appreciating the need for sleep

If you're like most parents, you spent a ton of time and energy (and often money) to get your baby to sleep. But for some reason, getting your older child to sleep has become less of a priority. I'd argue your child needs help with sleep throughout their childhood, even through the teen years.

If you can prioritize only one thing in this chapter, choose sleep. It's the most powerful mental health buffer.

Here's why: Sleep is vital to whole body wellness. During sleep, the brain and body are both resting and working at the same time. Without enough sleep, the body doesn't function at its best. Table 13-1 details the important things that happen when kids do, or do not, sleep well.

If you wonder what you can do to help strengthen your kids' immunity, skip the "immune building" supplements and encourage more sleep. Restorative sleep is vital to a functioning immune system, and kids who get less sleep are at greater risk of illness.

TABLE 13-1 Sleep Consequences in Children

Body or Brain Function	With Optimal Sleep	With Poor Sleep
Learning and memory	The brain strengthens newly acquired information, transferring it from short-term to long-term storage, which is crucial for learning.	Sleep deprivation is linked to deficits in attention, problem-solving, impulse control, and working memory.
Brain growth	Unused neural connections are eliminated and important ones are reinforced, optimizing cognitive efficiency.	Poor sleep disrupts white and gray matter integrity, impairing communication between different brain regions, including the prefrontal cortex.
Body metabolism	Kids grow when they sleep. In addition, sleep regulates glucose metabolism and energy restoration, reducing the risk of obesity and insulin resistance.	Growth hormone secretion may be disrupted. Sleep deprivation alters glucose metabolism and disrupts appetite-regulating hormones.
Brain metabolism	During slow-wave sleep, the *glymphatic system,* a specialized waste clearance pathway in the central nervous system, removes metabolic waste.	Poor sleep leads to inefficient waste removal by the glymphatic system, affecting synaptic plasticity, working memory, attention, and executive function.
Emotional regulation	Sleep is essential to ensure proper function of the prefrontal cortex and amygdala.	Sleep disturbances deregulate stress hormones, alter serotonin function, heighten amygdala reactivity, and make the prefrontal cortex less active.
Immune function	Sleep enhances the function of infection-fighting cells and increases cytokine production.	Poor sleep compromises immune response, increasing susceptibility to infections.
Cardiovascular system	Heart rate and blood pressure decrease during deep sleep, allowing the cardiovascular system to rest and recover.	Poor sleep is associated with increased blood pressure variability and higher systemic inflammation markers.

Knowing that sleep impacts the whole family

Poor sleep can lead to emotional dysregulation, which can trigger behavioral and educational challenges that ripple through the entire household — when one kid isn't sleeping well, the whole family feels it.

Families deserve great sleep, yet too many parents believe years of poor sleep are unavoidable. They simply tolerate it because they feel like nothing can be done. This mindset leads to unhealthy habits and burnout. All parents deserve restorative, essential sleep — unapologetically and without feelings of guilt or selfishness. Period.

REMEMBER

Improving sleep in early and middle childhood can prevent compounding sleep issues during adolescence. Drastic sleep changes occur during the years of puberty, making preexisting sleep issues more difficult to improve.

SLEEP GUIDELINES FOR KIDS

Sleep duration and timing change rapidly in the first decade of life. In turn, generalized guidelines for sleep are unique for each age group. Currently, the American Academy of Sleep Medicine recommends the following sleep hours for kids:

- Ages 1–2 years: 11–14 total hours, including naps
- Ages 3–5 years: 10–13 total hours, including naps
- Ages 6–12 years: 9–12 hours
- Ages 13–18 years: 8–10 hours

It should be noted that little is known about sleep needs in children with neurodevelopmental conditions or other chronic medical issues. Sleep duration may also vary by race, ethnicity, culture, and environmental conditions.

Sleep changes throughout childhood are due to natural changes in sleep structure, melatonin secretion, and environmental factors. For more about melatonin and its role in sleep see Chapter 17.

Noting sleep differences in anxious kids

Sleep is essential to all kids, but it's *exceptionally* important for anxious kids. And here's the problem: Kids with anxiety don't sleep well. Sleep problems are pervasive in anxious kids, with up to 90 percent reporting at least one sleep difficulty including insomnia, nightmares, difficulty sleeping alone, fatigue, and reduced sleep hours. Plus, anxiety and sleep are intricately and bidirectionally linked. Anxiety leads to sleep issues, and sleep issues worsen anxiety.

TIP

Addressing sleep disorders is one way to help daytime anxiety symptoms. For more on common childhood sleep disorders and their treatments see Chapter 6.

As bedtime approaches, anxious kids may experience intrusive thoughts and heightened stress, which increases activity in the sympathetic nervous system (SNS) and elevates stress hormone levels. This makes it harder to fall asleep and decreases time in restorative REM sleep. Over time, repeated cycles of sleep struggle can lead to negative bedtime associations, avoidance, and increased parental dependence to fall asleep.

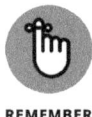

REMEMBER

Anxiety lives in a child's body and brain. Much of the stress they experience, day or night, requires you to be their proximate prefrontal cortex to help them gain control of their emotionally charged symptoms.

Bedsharing with anxious kids

Heightened fear and arousal around bedtime is common for kids with anxiety. What's also common? An exhausted, overwhelmed parent giving in to their anxious child's request to sleep in their bed.

Reactive bedsharing is co-sleeping with a child in response to a problem, not sharing a bed by choice. Allowing an anxious child to sleep in your bed ranks among the most frequent, counterproductive forms of parental *accommodation behaviors* among school-aged children with anxiety disorders.

Accommodation behaviors are the things parents do — like offering constant reassurance or changing routines — to help an anxious child feel better immediately, even if it reinforces the anxiety long term.

Recognizing the risks of bedsharing

Like the other accommodation behaviors I discuss in Chapter 12, bedsharing usually starts as an innocuous one-off event that seems natural, even pleasant. But repeating this pattern over time has consequences. Read Allison's story:

> Allison is a cautious, sensitive 6-year-old with mild separation anxiety. A few weeks ago, she woke up in the middle of the night, crying and afraid, saying she was scared of the dark and worried that something bad might happen. Her parents, exhausted and unsure of how to help, let Allison sleep in their bed for comfort that night.
>
> Since then, she asks to get in their bed every night, and it seems like her nighttime anxiety is worse. She's scared of her bed, and the bedtime routine is a battle. She cries, begs, and repeatedly comes out of her room, making the nights unbearable.
>
> Now Allison's parents are losing sleep, they have no time together as a couple, and they are exhausted. Plus, they feel guilty that the once-peaceful bedtime routine is now something they resent. They just want Allison to sleep in her own bed again, but they don't know what to do.

Bedsharing creates a nasty cycle that's hard to break. It starts with letting your anxious child sleep in bed with you *once.* Then, subsequent nights start by them begging and pleading to do it again. Eventually, this begging routine becomes a bedtime expectation. Your child's nervous system ramps up to fight the bedtime battle, increasing their stress hormone levels. And since they are physically hyper-alert, sleep becomes fragmented, leading to fatigue and irritability the following day. Rinse and repeat.

WARNING

Reactive bedsharing isn't offering the comfort or relief that you think it is. This type of persisting accommodation is associated with more *prolonged* anxious behavior and *increased* nighttime symptoms. Bedsharing in school-aged children is associated with higher rates of bedtime resistance, nighttime fears, night wakings, nightmares, daytime sleepiness, and clinical problems like separation anxiety, hyperactivity, and oppositionality.

If you want to stop bedsharing, know that breaking the cycle requires planning and dedication to the process — there are no quick fixes. Evidence suggests combining gradual exposure, consistent routines, and parental boundary-setting until your child has grown accustomed to sleeping alone. For more details on these approaches see Chapter 17.

Seeing when bedsharing may be okay

It's important to distinguish reactive bedsharing from *intentional bedsharing,* or when co-sleeping is proactively chosen due to personal preference or cultural norms. Intentional bedsharing can be done well when it's a strategic family choice — all of the kids are over 1 year old, there's space for everyone to sleep comfortably, everyone wakes up rested, and the kids are able to sleep independently when needed.

WARNING

Bedsharing with infants under the age of 1 is associated with suffocation and sudden infant death syndrome. It is not recommended by the American Academy of Pediatrics under any circumstances.

Committing to healthy bedtime habits

The best way to deal with sleep problems is to prevent them in the first place. I know, easier said than done. Here I offer you some foundational evidence-supported bedtime habits. Some are simple, not all are easy — but the health of you and your family is worth these efforts.

Choose great sleep for yourself

I'm putting this on the top of the list for a reason. Some yawn-filled days are unavoidable, but chronic fatigue directly impacts a parent's own health, daytime productivity, and quality of parenting efforts. Sleep experts suggest that adults need 7-9 hours of sleep for optimal functioning.

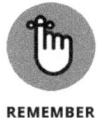

Parental stress negatively impacts childhood sleep patterns. Prioritizing your own sleep improves your ability to encourage great sleep for your child.

Build an environment for sleep success

A child's bedroom is for sleeping, and it needs to be built for that purpose. Keep the room dark, cool, cozy, and — most importantly — screen-free. Limit distracting items, like toys, games, and decor, until sleeping improves.

Plan a bedtime routine and stick to it

Having a consistent routine helps kids fall asleep by creating positive sleep associations. Choose a sequence of soothing activities that can be conducted in the same order each night and in various locations, like on vacation or at Grandma's house.

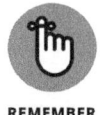

Routines are reliable and predictable, not rigid. It's the consistent sequence of events that makes a routine helpful, although each step may have subtle variation from night to night.

A great bedtime routine should last about 15 minutes. If your routine lasts more than an hour or has escalated to 22 steps, then it's an accommodation behavior that needs to be changed.

Determine sleep placement

Often a child's natural circadian rhythm conflicts with environmental factors like work and sport schedules, family activities and events, school and daycare start times, weekend activities, and more. Best practice is to create and defend parent-determined bedtimes, even through the teen years. For more on circadian cycle development see Chapter 17.

Add calming techniques

Bedtime is a great time for practicing calming techniques, like meditation, guided imagery, progressive muscle relaxation, or deep belly breathing (see Chapter 16). These tools immediately decrease anxiety and promote rest, and incorporating them at bedtime is practice for when kids have to use them independently during times of daytime stress.

Keep screens out of the bedroom

REMEMBER

Never. Just don't. Digital media use is associated with later bedtimes and fewer sleep hours. Research suggests screens interfere with sleep by increasing light exposure, psychological alertness, and displacement of time that could be spent sleeping. Screens in bed aren't great for anyone — consider your own bedtime screen habits, too! Find more about screen time later in this chapter.

Use a visual schedule

TIP

For younger kids, a visual chart or diagram can remind your child of what is necessary and what to expect. Extra stories? Not on the chart. Not on the chart? Not going to be done. Be amenable to appropriate requests, but limit your attention to unnecessary or anxiety-driven asks.

Bring out the teddy bear

Studies have found transition objects can reduce bedtime stress and reinforce positive sleep-association skills for all ages. If your child has a favorite teddy bear or lovey, include it in the bedtime routine.

TIP

Typical electronic sleep tracking devices can be helpful to monitor general sleep trends. However, due to the large variability in sleep needs and lack of extensive testing in children, much of the data available on a typical sleep tracking device (an Apple watch or a camera system, for example) has little correlation with sleep quality or efficacy.

Expect variability

Even with exceptional structure and routine, not every night will be perfect. Your child is an independent person with their own set of internal and external stressors that will change their bedtime experience from time to time.

Seek professional help if needed

If your efforts to improve your family's sleep aren't going as planned, look for a sleep medicine physician in your area. These doctors utilize extra years of training in sleep science to diagnose sleep disorders and create detailed plans for your family's specific needs. Often a referral is needed from your pediatrician for sleep medicine support. Reach out if you need help.

Moving for Mental Health

Have you ever experienced clarity of mind after a walk outside? Less anger after a strength session at the gym? Maybe you've noticed that your daily focus is better after working out in the morning? These social-emotional benefits of exercise are for kids, too!

Exercise is a powerful, natural way to manage anxiety and build emotional resilience. Movement decreases stress hormone levels and naturally boosts "feel-good hormones," like dopamine and serotonin. Exercise improves sleep and increases executive function and selective attention, leading to improved school performance. Group activities encourage social interaction and team-building. Plus, exercise is a great distractor, pulling a child's thoughts away from their worries.

TIP

Both strenuous exercise and anxiety create similar changes in the body, like increased heart rate, shortness of breath, and sweating. During exercise, repeated exposure to these physical changes, paired with satisfying and quick recovery, serves as a form of *extinction learning* — how the brain learns that a sensation or feeling is not a threat, helping to reduce the stress response over time.

Embracing the outdoors

Kids aren't meant to incubate under fluorescent and LED lights. They need to get outside to move their bodies and exercise their brains. Being in nature can have profound effects on mental wellness.

Studies show that spending just 20 minutes outside each day can

» Decrease stress, anxiety, and negative thinking and improve mood, self-esteem, and social connections

» Reduce aggression, depression, and feelings of isolation

» Lessen the impacts of negative events

» Improve focus in children with attention deficits

» Stimulate sensory integration

Being outside helps anxious kids. The natural environment is constantly moving and changing, with different tactile sensations, sights, smells, and sounds. Anxious kids attune to the environment more than to their inner worries and fears, giving them release from stress and anxiety symptoms. Plus, nature provides places to explore risk and physical limits.

Energizing family movement

Children ages 3–5 should be physically active most of the day through structured and unstructured play. Kids over age 6 should get sweaty for at least one hour of each day, seven hours per week. Encourage a mix of both aerobic and muscle strengthening work. The following are tips to help your family reach these goals:

» **There is no one exercise that's perfect for every person or everybody.** One kid may love basketball; another may excel at martial arts. Find an activity they enjoy, where they participate easily and have routine access. Choose things with room for challenge and growth, but recognize that if the activity is too hard, boring, or puts them at a disadvantage among their peers, they will be less likely to participate.

» **In young kids, the goal is fun.** This is the time to explore how their body moves and to determine which physical skills come more naturally than others. Early exercise shouldn't be about competition, future athletic performance, or getting a college athletic scholarship.

- **>> Try to avoid rewards for physical movement.** (I'm looking at you, "after-soccer-practice-treat-bag.") The reward for movement should be having one-on-one time with coaches and friends and making their brain and body feel better.

- **>> Daily movement doesn't have to be all in one session.** Multiple small efforts throughout the day may be more beneficial for some kids. Spend at least a few minutes every day outside — school gym classes and active recesses count.

- **>> Exercise is important for all kids.** Kids with different abilities and those with chronic medical conditions need movement, too. See the Appendix for exercise resources for all kids.

- **>> Defend recess in your child's school,** and support as many days for outside play as possible. Let your kids walk or bike to school when they can safely do so.

TIP

- **>> Thank a gym teacher.** Movement is so important to kids, yet physical education is often pushed aside for other academic pursuits. Physical education helps kids find out how they enjoy moving their bodies for long-term health.

- **>> Moms and dads move, too!** Time to dust off the treadmill, grab a yoga mat, or head outside for a walk. Show your child that moving your body feels great at any age and that staying active is a way to take responsibility for the healthy body you have.

Fueling the Anxious Body and Brain

Kids who struggle to eat a variety of whole, natural foods may be missing some essential nutrients required for healthy growth. *Essential nutrients* are elements and substrates that the body can't produce on its own and that must be obtained from the diet. If your child isn't eating food containing the essentials, they may not have the building blocks required for natural stress-reducing hormones.

A few of the essential nutrients strongly associated with mental health are B-complex vitamins, zinc, magnesium, fatty acids, vitamin D, and iron. Table 13-2 lists kid-friendly foods with these components. These essential nutrients and more are further detailed in Chapter 11.

TABLE 13-2   Essential Nutrients in Common Foods

Essential Nutrient	Food
B-complex vitamins	Avocados, whole-grain breads and pasta, fortified milk and cereals, eggs, lean turkey and chicken, hummus, refried beans, peanut or almond butter
Zinc	Lean beef, chicken, turkey, and pork; egg yolks; cashew butter; shellfish
Magnesium	Leafy greens, legumes, nuts, seeds, whole grains, dark chocolate, brown rice, bananas, avocado, potatoes with skin, berries, tofu
Fatty acids	Salmon, trout, eggs, fortified dairy, chia seeds, almond or peanut butter, edamame
Vitamin D	Fortified dairy products and cereals, fatty fish, egg yolks
Iron	Lean meats, eggs, fortified cereals and oatmeal, spinach, dried fruits, beans, broccoli, peas

WARNING

Whole nuts and small seeds are choking hazards for kids under age 5. Generally speaking, kids shouldn't eat whole nuts until they can spell the word N-U-T-S. Until then, use nut butters or powders as alternatives.

TIP

Growing brains and nervous systems need fat. Generally speaking, young kids don't need foods commercially labeled as "low fat," unless specifically recommended by your pediatrician.

Connecting anxiety and food issues

Young children with anxiety often struggle to meet nutritional goals. They may avoid unfamiliar foods, stick to a narrow range of "safe" foods, or be sensitive to textures, colors, or smells. Stress hormones can disrupt hunger cues, leading to irregular eating patterns. Some anxious kids will overeat to self-soothe, and others may lose their appetite.

REMEMBER

Anxiety itself can manifest as stomachaches, nausea, or other tummy issues (see Chapter 6), making eating physically uncomfortable.

In addition, stressful meal environments influence how an anxious child eats. At home, well-meaning adults may pressure children to eat, which can heighten stress and further reduce appetite. Children may worry about eating "wrong" or about others' opinions during mealtimes. At school, the cafeteria may be an anxiety-triggering place, making kids eat quickly, if at all.

REMEMBER

Nutritional deficits are more important in kids who are genetically vulnerable to mood disorders. Not all bodies require the same foods or utilize nutritional components equally.

Making small changes

REMEMBER

As science continues to find out more about the relationship between anxiety and nutrition, you have the power to make small changes in your food buying and mealtime habits today.

I emphasize *small* changes because change is hard. Nutrient-dense foods can be costly and tough to find. Routine mealtimes require families to dance around work schedules, after-school activities, and social obligations. Food allergies and other medical conditions may limit options. And not everyone knows how to or likes to cook. For the following reasons and more, every family's nutritional journey is unique.

TIP

If and when you feel ready make changes to improve your family's nutrition, turn to the following suggestions. Can only do one? Pick the first one.

>> **Eat more dinners together as a family, at home, and without screens.** Offer what you feel is a healthy,

balanced meal, but keep your mealtimes positive times of connection with less direct focus on what your child is or is not eating. Meanwhile, enjoy a variety of foods on your own plate to model diverse and joyful eating.

>> **Involve kids in meal planning and preparation.** This is a great way to find new favorites.

>> **Eat slowly.** Fast-paced mealtimes and on-the-go eating don't allow kids to develop feelings of satisfaction or fullness.

>> **Read the labels.** Choose food items with shorter ingredient lists, reducing exposure to non-nutritive additives, dyes, refined sugars and oils, and preservatives. Choose dye-free medications, and ask your pharmacist whether there are dye-free prescription options for any medications your child may take.

>> **Build a healthier grocery list.** Consider less processed meats, and prioritize fresh or frozen fruits and vegetables. Limit carbonated, caffeinated, and high-calorie beverages.

>> **Cook and store smartly.** Use glass dishware to store food and reheat items in the microwave. Wash plastic dishware and water bottles by hand to avoid the dishwasher's high heat.

Succeeding with Screen Time

Screens are everywhere. You need them, your kids love them, and we're all affected by them. To be clear, I'm not anti-screens — we live in a digital ecosystem with inherent conveniences and benefits. But this book is about anxious kids. That's why it's essential to understand how screens uniquely affect anxious kids — and why we need to use them wisely.

WARNING

Navigating the headlines that make claims for and against screen time can cause any parent whiplash. However, decades of screen research have revealed a few consistent truths:

>> **Excessive screen time is bad for your kid.** The more
screen time a child has, the more likely the negative
effects, some of which can be profound. Excessive screen
time is associated with significant learning, language, and
social-emotional delays in young kids, which are carried
though early and middle childhood. Screen time can also
lead to physical issues like changes to eye development,
obesity, oral cavities, headaches, and repetitive
use injuries.

>> **Not all screen time carries the same risk.** Television
viewing, computer use, video gaming, social media, big
screens, little screens, screens together, screens alone,
boys and screens, girls and screens . . . these variations
create unique risk factors, and not all kids respond to the
same screen time in the same way. However, the consistent theme is less screen time helps protect kids from
negative effects.

>> **Too much screen time interferes with emotional
development.** This includes delays in emotional compre-
hension, increased emotional dysregulation, and increased
aggressive behavior. The effects have been shown to last
months after excessive exposure, increasing concerns that
excessive screen time is creating changes in brain
development.

>> **Social skill development is hindered by screens.** Using
digital tools to communicate, rather than navigating an
in-person interaction, potentially reinforces avoidance
behaviors and worsens social anxiety. Like all avoidance
behaviors I discuss in Chapter 12, when kids escape to the
digital world, they miss out on real-life opportunities to
practice being a social human.

>> **Screens foster emotional avoidance.** Getting lost in a
YouTube video is a lot easier than facing an uncomfortable
emotion. This short-term relief from discomfort reinforces
a child's need to calm down using screens, reduces their
tolerance for discomfort, and robs them of the opportunity
to work through an emotion on their own. Over time, kids
can develop a reliance on screens for emotional control.

>> **Screen time displaces protective buffers.** Screens take away from time spent in areas of life that protect against anxiety's effects, like sleeping or exercising. When that happens, screen time's negative effects are amplified.

Acknowledging interference

Screens interfere with your parenting. I know, this one stings a little bit. Hear me out.

Parental technoference is the term used to describe how your relationship with your kids is influenced by your technology use. Exploring the consequences of this relational change and technology-driven disconnect from our children's lives is a new area of emerging research, and early results are a bit sobering. Just like your kids, you're affected by the screen in your hand more than you know or care to admit.

The single most important factor that supports a child's healthy social-emotional development is consistent and supportive parent-child interactions. Screens interfere with this work in multiple ways. Parental technoference reduces a parent's ability to pay attention, be responsive, and display emotional warmth. Additionally, multitasking with devices makes it more difficult to respond to your child's cues and manage difficult child behavior.

Technoference increases a child's anxiety and behavioral challenges. When parents use their phones during interactions with their children, researchers see higher rates of whining, tantrums, and aggression. Children may act out more to get attention, even if that attention is negative. Parents distracted by screens are less patient and are more likely to react harshly to misbehavior. Kids, in turn, become more frustrated when parents are physically present but emotionally unavailable.

REMEMBER

Not using your phone around your child is not realistic, nor the point of this section. Rather, I want to recognize the reality of the challenges of parental screen use and emphasize the idea that it's not just the kids' screen time that deserves reflective evaluation.

Constructing safer screen time at home

I know you've already heard a million suggestions on how to manage screen time. But unlike before, you now have a new framework to help you understand the importance of helping your anxious kid with screens. With that in mind, review the following screen time tips:

>> **Create non-negotiable, screen-free boundaries today.** Like, right now. In my house, boundaries include no screens in the bedroom or bathroom, and no screens at the dinner table. Remember, boundaries also include places screens *can* be, like on the living room couch or in the family office. Be clear about where screens can and can't be used.

>> **Reach family goals first, then allow screens.** Decide on the activities your child must do daily. Maybe that's homework, chores, sports or music practice, playing outside, or family activity time. Spend your energy defending and protecting the good stuff — if there's time left over, let screen time be okay.

>> **Make screen time routine.** Part of the reason kids get obsessed with screens is due to their sporadic availability. Just like success on a slot machine, kids get hyper-focused to try, try, try to get more screen time when the reward is inconsistent. If screen time is routinely part of the day, it carries less weight of importance and extinguishes the drive created by intermittent reinforcement.

>> **Remember that less is better.** For young kids, keep recreational screen time to less than one hour per day, less than two hours for school-aged kids. (Remember these amounts are weekly averages, not strict 24-hour goals.) Limiting time takes effort on your part, but don't feel like you have to be a cruise director. Let your child figure out what they want to do in their safe play spaces. And it's okay for them to be bored.

>> **Choose better content.** When screens are on, choose shows, games, and sites with quality content. Block apps and services that you prefer your child not use.

>> **Use parental restrictions and turn off auto-play.** Simple parental restrictions are included with most devices and

operating systems. If you purchase a device for your child, take a minute to learn how to use parental controls to keep your kid stay safe while meeting time or content goals. Turning off auto-play helps to create breaks naturally where activities can be transitioned.

>> **Protect kids from stressful events.** Heavy-hitting and emotional news headlines are now the norm, and young kids don't need to know the details of every tragic news story. When significant news is breaking, take extra care to control the content.

>> **Avoid using screens as reward or punishment.** This makes screens seem more valuable than they are.

>> **Be fully present.** Time with your kids is based on quality, not quantity. Don't let screens get in the way of the few minutes you may be able to connect. Turn on the "Do Not Disturb" mode on your devices during before- and after-school times. If you need to check your phone, be clear about your intent, like "I'm sending a quick email to my boss, then I'm all yours."

>> **Limit the number of screens in your home.** Young kids don't need their own device. The more screens you have, the more work it is to monitor or track usage. Let generous relatives know your stance before gift-giving seasons.

>> **Watch your own use.** Protect yourself from the negative effects of screens by being mindful of your own habits. Remember that kids are watching what you do all the time, so be a living example of how screens can support healthy relationships.

You have the power to reduce the negative effects of screens; your kids can't do this on their own. From toddlers to teens, the only consistent way to reduce screen time is for adults to take specific actions to limit it, which also means creating limits on screen time for ourselves, too.

REMEMBER

You're the leader of your home, and you have to lead by example — hard truth, right? We can't tell our kids to "go play" if we won't play with them. We can't expect our "picky eater" to eat their veggies when there's nothing green on our plates. And we can't plan on them happily obliging to turn off their video game when we have one eye on our own phone.

Prioritizing Play

Renowned child psychologist Jean Piaget is attributed with saying, "Play is the work of childhood." This sentiment reflects the importance of allowing time for the serious matter of play.

Play is full of complexities and benefits that are engrained in developmental growth and progress. Kids play before they speak, play before they walk — it's that important for proper development. For anxious kids, play can be a valuable respite from the stress of their world, while equally being an activity that defends their mental wellness.

Balancing types of play

There are two broad categories of play: structured and unstructured. Both types of play are essential for a child's development, but they offer different benefits and challenges. A healthy balance between the two is ideal for promoting cognitive, social, emotional, and physical growth.

» **Structured play happens within the defined rules of the adult world.** It is organized, with goals, limits, and guidance. Structured play includes playing board games, following LEGO instructions, and participating in rule-based role-playing games. It also includes the things you sign your kids up for: the dance classes, the piano lessons, and the youth sports teams (see Chapter 14). The goals of structured play are skill development, discipline, and focus.

» **Unstructured play helps anxious kids.** It is child-directed, open-ended, and requires imagination. Kids are doing unstructured play when they invent stories, play store, build forts, draw rainbow unicorns, play tag, and make slime. Unstructured play encourages creativity and experimentation in a place where there are no rules or goals. This type of play provides emotional relief, encourages self-expression, and reduces stress.

REMEMBER

Play is normal, important, healthy, and powerful. All types of play are beneficial, and this applies to all from babies to big kids. When children enjoy the benefits of both play types, they avoiding the downsides of too much structure or too little guidance.

Valuing play for anxious kids

Play is the antidote to anxiety. Independent, unstructured play is a time to foster calculated risk-taking, push limits, promote self-confidence, and build self-esteem.

Play is a protective stress buffer. Physical activity releases endorphins, boosts mood, and lowers stress hormones. Play teaches resilience by allowing children to fail and try again in a low-pressure context, helping them to manage frustration and anxiety more effectively. Play also helps kids cope with adverse experiences, decreasing the impact of environmental stress.

Play promotes social-emotional development by helping children learn essential skills to work though conflict, build problem-solving skills, and practice leadership. The back-and-forth structure of play strengthens relational skills and improves emotional intelligence.

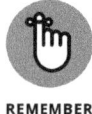
REMEMBER

Play is a great distractor. It allows kids to take a break from the constant pressure — often created by us — to achieve and better themselves. Play is a place where there are no mistakes, the worries of the day are gone, and they can enjoy the present moment.

Avoiding overscheduling

Exposure to new hobbies and organized activities is a luxury for many children, but being constantly scheduled as a young child increases the risk for burnout as a teen. Meanwhile, constant enrollment in activities creates the trap that your child depends on you for entertainment all the time.

Kids need space for unstructured play. Let young kids explore their own interests through one to two hours daily of free, self-directed play. Create screen-free spaces. Provide open-ended toys and craft supplies from things you find around the house. Locate safe outdoor play spaces. And leave room for messes.

Generally speaking, kids don't have to be in any organized activities until kindergarten. As kids get older, schedule no more than one hour of organized activity per week per their age. For example, a 7-year-old should not have more than seven hours of scheduled activities per week.

Leaning into Routines

Anxiety thrives under uncertainty and chaos. Routines are the remedy. They help anxious kids because their consistency builds habits without adding pressure or strict time demands. In addition, a few daily routines add stability to the natural changes of life, helping kids feel grounded and safe when things get stressful.

Distinguishing routines from schedules

Don't confuse a routine with a schedule. Routines are anticipated and purposeful, with some flexibility. In contrast, a schedule is a sequence of planned activities with specific, fixed times. Although similar constructs, routines hold two elements that provide better support for development:

>> **Routines are predictable but not rigid.** They prioritize the *order* of expected events rather than exact timing. For example, bedtime and dinner routines each have sequential elements, but the timing may vary daily. Research shows that these predictable moments buffer the impact of stress on mental health.

>> **Routines provide a high level of accessibility.** Participating in the same sequence of steps builds mastery and confidence over time. For example, kids can help set the table at dinnertime or choose their own book to read with a parent at bedtime.

Here's the important part: It's not just about the work of the day, it's also about you! Children benefit from predicable *relationships* and parents who behave in predictable ways. Kids need parents whose response, attention, and support are reliable, available, and expected. This includes having consistent expectations and behavior management strategies. Predictability and accessibility are foundational for secure attachment, feelings of safety, and maintaining trust.

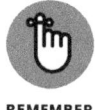

Children don't need perfect parents; they need predictable parents.

Building home routines

Routines don't have to be complicated. Routines are simply everyday tasks, organized into a consistent, manageable sequence of steps. Use the following suggestions to help make routines work:

>> **Pick a flexible time of day.** This allows time for practice. Your child may feel less rushed setting the table before dinner versus completing a morning routine before school.

>> **Use visual aids.** Help your child remember multistep routines by using pictures or checklists. Offer positive reinforcement for all the tasks completed independently.

>> **Allow your child to add their input.** They may have opinions on which things should be included or an order they prefer.

>> **Include daily chores.** Chores strengthen executive functioning skills, including time management and organization. They teach the value of being in a family and improve self-esteem. Plus, it's one way to instill responsibility and teach life skills, while feeling the satisfaction of success.

>> **Create weekly routines, too.** Taco Tuesdays, Sunday church services, and Saturday movie nights are all stress-buffers, too. In addition, routines connecting children to previous generations may be particularly impactful.

Kids are able to have daily, age-appropriate chores beginning at age 3. As a general suggestion, give them one chore per year of age.

Chapter **14**

Thriving in School and Sports for Anxious Kids

Young kids spend most of their waking hours at school and organized activities. All kids deserve healthy support in these places. Thankfully, children often tell us what they need to succeed. We just need to listen.

In this chapter, you find out about the spectrum of anxiety for kids at school and ways to help. This chapter also discusses sports participation, highlighting the benefits and risks of organized sports, introducing the signs of sports anxiety, and offering ways to help keep your athlete having fun on the field.

Expecting Back-to-School Anxiety

Back-to-school anxiety is exceptionally common. Kids can express nervousness, a change in sleep behaviors, and even mild physical symptoms during the first few weeks of the academic year. Many other types of school transitions can cause similar stress, such as a starting at a new school, returning after a long vacation, or going back after a favorite classmate has moved away.

TIP

Most kids will adjust to their new classroom within a few weeks. As always, your child's educators are prepared to help. In addition, here are a few ways to help your child from home:

» **Do practice visits.** Gradually expose your child to the school and their teacher. Take a tour. Visit the classroom. Introduce them to the principal. Walk them through their schedule. Play on the playground. Bring them with you to ask a question at the office, practicing a drop-off on the way. Find opportunities for repetition and exposure to get them comfortable.

» **Listen to their concerns.** Let them express their worries, and validate their concerns. Use this time to game-plan how they'll handle concerning situations. These conversations don't have to be long and formal; just a quick check-in will do.

» **Lean into your routines.** Use your established routines (see Chapter 13) to make sure your child eats a balanced diet, moves every day, and gets enough sleep.

» **Communicate with the school.** Educators have extensive experience in providing support to their students. Let the teacher know your child is having some difficulty, and see what can be done to help them have better days. Consider supports such as a warm hand-off in the morning, some extra downtime, or other positive reinforcement techniques.

» **Stay calm and positive.** Let your demeanor and tone reflect confidence. Talk through your own feelings and how you're coping. Model calming techniques, and let your child join in. Encourage social interactions and confidence-building activities outside of school.

REMEMBER

Kids don't tell you they are feeling anxious; they show you.

Experiencing Anxiety in School

Outside of normal transitional anxiety, school can be a source of anxiety itself. School can also be the first place symptoms present. Here's Lisa's story:

> Lisa is a bright and creative second grader. She enjoys school and has no trouble making new friends. But after a fun and relaxing summer, she is having a hard time getting to school in the morning.
>
> For the first few weeks of school, Lisa seemed more irritable and had more difficulty falling asleep. Additionally, she asked daily to FaceTime her best friend who moved to a different school over the summer. Her parents attributed these changes to busier days at school and simply wanting to catch up with her friend.
>
> During the first parent-teacher conference, Lisa's teacher mentioned that she's doing well academically but appears distracted in class and no longer participates in her reading group. The teacher also revealed that Lisa is asking to go to the nurse's office before every afternoon recess — information unknown to her parents.
>
> After the conference, Lisa's parents asked her about school and her teacher's comments. Lisa became visibly distressed. She says she doesn't like being called on by the teacher and is worried about making mistakes. Then she became tearful and asked her parents if she could be homeschooled.

Lisa's experience isn't uncommon. For kids with anxiety triggered by the school experience, concerning signs are exceptionally subtle or nonexistent at home. It's often the teachers and school counselors who bring the issue to the parent's attention.

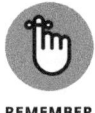

REMEMBER

If a teacher, coach, or other trusted care provider suggests that your child may be showing signs of a mental health issue, take it seriously. Especially if your child's symptoms are situational, you may never see a warning sign. It takes a village!

Identifying school anxiety

For kids experiencing school anxiety, symptoms may include the following:

>> Feeling the need to check in with their parents throughout the school day, using their phones or computers

>> Squirming in their seat and not paying attention, often triggering concern for attention-deficit/hyperactivity disorder (ADHD)

>> Asking to go to the nurse's office for stomachaches, headaches, or other ailments

>> Showing aggression in the classroom, like attacking another child or a teacher, throwing things, or pushing over a desk

>> Being overly self-critical, leading to missing or late assignments because the work isn't perfect

>> Delaying the morning routine, with more tantrums, refusal to get ready, or physical complaints in attempts to stay at home

REMEMBER

School anxiety isn't an anxiety diagnosis in itself; rather it's a symptom of many types of anxiety conditions. Getting a full evaluation helps you better understand what's really going on with your child. For more about the diagnostic assessment see Chapter 8.

Supporting anxious kids in the classroom

Educators are prepared to identify and support anxiety in their students. For most kids, communication with the school and your child's educators will be enough to initiate needed plans. However, when your child's anxiety is severe enough to impact their ability to learn, formal accommodations, like 504s and Individualized Education Programs (IEPs), may be needed.

>> **A 504 Plan is designed for students who have a disability that substantially limits learning.** It falls under Section 504 of the Rehabilitation Act of 1973, which is a civil rights law ensuring that students with disabilities have equal access to education. Developed by a team of educators, counselors,

and administrators, a 504 plan provides accommodations to help your child manage anxiety in school without changing what your child is expected to learn.

>> **An IEP is a more intensive support plan for students whose anxiety significantly impacts their ability to learn and make progress in school.** It falls under the Individuals with Disabilities Education Act (IDEA) and provides both accommodations and specialized instruction. An IEP requires a full learning and psychological evaluation performed by a trained clinician. These plans include specific learning goals and may include counseling, social skills training, and small-group instruction.

REMEMBER

Accommodations aren't a treatment, or a "crutch," for anxiety. They are meant to be temporary aids to students while they progress through their treatment. As students' anxiety symptoms get under control, teachers can alter and/or remove classroom accommodations entirely.

If you believe your child needs a 504 Plan or IEP, ask for a school evaluation. In most cases, you can initiate this process with a formal request letter. After the evaluation, the school will meet with you to review the results and, if eligible, develop an individualized plan. Find resources about academic accommodations in the Appendix.

Refusing to Go to School

Providing students with support in the classroom and school can minimize stress for students with anxiety and help prevent school refusal (SR) behaviors. The following is Andrea's experience:

About two months ago, Andrea, a healthy 11-year-old, complained of a stomachache before school. Thinking it was stomach flu, her parents allowed her to stay home. During that day at home, she quickly perked up, wanting to run errands and play video games. Now, attending school has become a constant battle.

Mornings have turned chaotic. Andrea complains of stomach-aches, nausea, dizziness, and headaches — often crying, refusing to get dressed, or screaming that she "can't go." When her parents insist she leave, she's slammed doors, thrown her backpack, and locked herself in the bathroom.

At school, she frequently visits the nurse and has been sent home early multiple times. Her frustration is visible — crying at recess, walking out of math, and ending up in the principal's office on two separate occasions in the past month.

Understanding school refusal

Anxiety leads to avoidance behaviors, and SR is a severe and complex type of avoidance. SR is not a psychiatric diagnosis, but kids with SR commonly have primary diagnoses of anxiety or mood-related disorders. SR often arises during transition points such as moving from primary to secondary school.

Kids with SR strongly resist attending school, displaying excessive fear, unhappiness, or unexplained physical symptoms that lead to school absenteeism that parents are aware of. In some cases, they experience chronic emotional distress, such as persistent sadness or sleep disturbances, which significantly disrupt regular attendance.

Multiple factors drive school absences related to SR, including anxiety-related stress, stress-induced physical symptoms that limit participation, and sensory overload that causes emotional shutdowns. Various emotional and behavioral conditions, such as low self-concept, cyberbullying, and excessive technology use, can increase the risk of SR.

Helping a child with school refusal

Encouraging routine school attendance for kids with SR requires an expert-driven, comprehensive plan. The plan should include interventions for the child directly, their family, and their educators. The following describes this level of support:

>> **Collaboration with the school team:** As soon as your child starts avoiding or missing school, notify the school for

support. Schools often need to implement a structured, step-by-step plan to help students stay for the full day. This plan may include unique morning transition strategies, peer mentor connections, increased break times, or temporary workload modifications to prevent shutdowns.

>> **Professional emotional and behavioral support:** Kids with SR need evidence-supported counseling or therapy, such as cognitive behavioral therapy (CBT) or dialectical behavioral therapy (DBT), to develop emotional regulation and coping strategies (see Chapter 9).

>> **Social support:** Encourage small, structured social opportunities at school and in the community to help rebuild connections. Additionally, explore extracurricular activities in which your child may feel more comfortable engaging.

Looking at the Landscape of Today's Youth Sports

For millions of families, the rhythm of life is dictated by two things: the academic calendar and the organized sports calendar. After-school practices, games, coaching sessions, and skills camps dominate the extracurricular calendar, with kids beginning to participate at younger ages every year.

The following sections describe the benefits your child can receive from organized sports and the potential sports-related anxiety a child can face.

Reaping the benefits of organized sports

Organized youth sports can offer significant benefits to kids. Sports participation promotes mental and physical development, higher activity levels, and better overall health. Sports enhance physical skills like hand-eye coordination, movement, and strength and also fostering academic, self-regulation, and life skills.

TIP

Determining when to start organized sports is unique to every family. Generally speaking, most kids have the basic physical ability and interest after the age of 6.

Receiving the benefits of youth sport participation is highly dependent on two things: the environment created by the coaches and organization around them, and your expectation and support of their participation.

REMEMBER

Youth sports — even for the youngest ages — have become a highly organized business industry. Club sports sell the illusion of elite status and college scholarships, but they also increase the risk of burnout in the very athletes they promise to help succeed — especially when children are encouraged to participate beyond their physical readiness or unrealistic expectations are placed on their performance. Being fully aware of this paradox is important as your child begins to participate.

Early sports participation is best supported by healthy parent-child relationships. As privileged and talented as young athletes are, parental over-involvement in a child's athletic career can lead to decreased player enjoyment and negative player behaviors. Supporting the positive aspects of hard work, follow-through on commitments, and good sportsmanship are shown to be associated with increased motivation for athlete participation and a better relationship with parents.

Examining anxiety in organized sports

Sports participation and physical activity are beneficial to the mental health of young kids, even serving as an effective part of a comprehensive anxiety treatment plan. Sports improve emotional regulation by teaching kids to manage frustration, handle mistakes, and overcome setbacks. Compared to exercise alone, participation in organized sports is associated with a decreased risk of anxiety and depression, reduced stress, increased self-esteem, and improved social abilities. However, not all sports impact mental health in the same way.

Individual sports provide the physical benefits of exercise, self-esteem development, and immense feelings of accomplishment. Unlike team sports, however, individual sports often come with increased anxiety due to the tendency to set intense personal goals, the pressure to differentiate themselves, and the constant pursuit of perfection and approval. Individual sport athletes, including gymnasts, figure skaters, and dancers, correlate with the highest level of anxiety in elite athletics.

Of course, kids with anxiety successfully participate in individual sports all the time. Recognizing that kids in individual sports can feel more pressure helps parents step in early if signs of problems arise. Focusing on fun, personal growth, and open communication goes a long way in helping them stay resilient, confident, and emotionally healthy.

Especially for kids in individual sports, strengthening habits that buffer against anxiety's impact, like sleep, family meals, and unstructured play, should be top of mind. For more details see Chapter 13.

Supporting Your Young Athlete

We've all seen the parent going nuts on the sidelines, arguing with refs, and coaching their child from the stands. These enthusiastic parents love their kids and are trying to show positive support. But supporting your athlete without being over-involved requires walking a very thin line.

Your healthy perspective with your child's early sports participation is critical to prevent early dropout and nurture a lifelong, healthy relationship with sports. The following are some ways to support your child as they begin organized sport participation.

Keeping the fun in sport

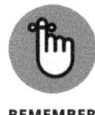

Sports are a game. Games are meant to be fun. That's it. So don't take youth sports so seriously. Early sports involvement is to find favorites, discover new skills, practice teamwork, and enjoy body movement. If your child's experience starts to shift away from the joy of play, then you're missing the point.

Encouraging physical literacy

Physical literacy is the ability, confidence, and motivation to be active throughout life. It requires fundamental movement skills, like running, jumping, throwing, catching, and balancing. Participating in organized sports is one opportunity to develop and refine these skills, but it's not the primary way kids learn movement.

TIP

Kids don't need organized sports to develop physical literacy. Model movement in your home and allow your kids to join in. Support physical activity classes in schools. Give kids time outdoors for unstructured play. All these things build a lifelong love of movement and a desire for a more active lifestyle.

Choosing variety as long as you can

A concerning trend in youth sports is *early specialization* — intensely focusing on one sport year-round and giving up others. Although beneficial in sports like gymnastics, diving, and figure skating, early specialization often leads to more injuries and a higher risk of burnout. In addition, kids who start intense training early limit extracurricular activities, have less unstructured play, and are more likely to drop out.

TIP

Athletic development happens by practicing a variety of movements and techniques. Young kids should play and explore many types of athletic activities throughout the year, including both team and individual efforts. For most sports, specialization doesn't need to happen until the teenage years.

Prioritizing recovery

The American Academy of Pediatrics recommends one day of rest per week and two to three months off from participation in any specific sport. The months don't have to be consecutive, but whenever you can, take these breaks in one-month increments during the year.

REMEMBER

Taking time off from a preferred sport does not mean becoming a couch potato. Staying active in other ways will help maintain conditioning and work on additional skills.

Sleep and nutrition are vitally important for athletic recovery and directly related to athletic performance. For more information see Chapter 13.

Modeling emotional control

When parents and coaches support emotional balance, they create a motivating environment that keeps kids active, engaged, and resilient. In turn, emotionally supported athletes who enjoy what they play are more likely to stay involved, forming friendships and positive emotional bonds.

REMEMBER

The foundation of your parent-child relationship in the context of sports is formed in the early years of participation. Know what kind of sports parent you want to be, and how you want to encourage a heathy relationship with sport in your child.

Handling the car ride home

Memories of countless games and tournaments come and go, and highlight reels get dusty. What's remembered are the hours and hours you spend in the car with your young athlete. Make the car ride home a positive space, and give your athlete great memories of this time spent together. The following are a few suggestions:

>> **Keep the game on the field, not in the car.** Your child knows when they have performed well or poorly, and they've likely already heard about it from their coach. Crank up some fun music. Talk about what's happening next. If your athlete brings up the game, be a reactive listener. Listen, don't fix. Focus the conversation on the big picture and not the outcome. Then, move on to a different topic.

TIP

If you must talk about the game, choose wisely. The only unsolicited comments about the performance are those that reflect the fun of sport, success of a new skill, and teamwork. This approach prevents your athlete from becoming hyper-focused on winning or making mistakes. The following are examples:

- "I loved watching you celebrate with your team after the first quarter."

- "You should feel proud of yourself that you kept going, even when it got tough."
- "Your routine looked great today — how did it feel to you?"
- "You really helped the coach by grabbing all the equipment after the game. That was a great way to be a helpful teammate."

TIP

If your child has been rude, unsportsmanlike, disrespectful, or has broken rules about spitting, cussing, or illegal play, you need to initiate the conversation about the game immediately. Describe what you saw, future expectations, and consequences for repeated negative behaviors.

>> **Maintain positivity always.** Focusing on your child's specific effort or performance, while they are feeling vulnerable or unsteady, creates resentment and unhappy silence. Talk to them the way you want them to talk to themselves. You're building the internal monologue that they will use in future tough moments.

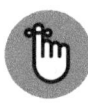

REMEMBER

Kids are learning how to contextualize athletics in their life by how you value and prioritize their sports experience. They are looking to your words, actions, and behaviors to determine what role athletics should take today and in their future.

>> **Praise the effort, not the outcome.** Don't guide your conversation based on "results." A kid can win the game but play without character. A loss can give an opportunity to try a new skill. The outcome isn't their identity.

REMEMBER

Your child's teammates are often their friends and classmates. Talking negatively about any other player has the power to change off-field relationships.

>> **Practice the 24-hour rule.** Your child needs space and time to digest the game and recover physically and emotionally — and you do too. By taking some time away from the event, both you and your child can separate the emotionality of the moment from the action that took place, leading to a space of more productive conversation about strategies to improve or decisions that need to be made.

>> **Sweet treats are for wins and losses.** A stop for ice cream or a special dinner treat can be a time to bond, but don't base special stops on performance. A surprise detour for a treat can celebrate life's small victories as equally as it can lift sprits after a defeat.

Teaming Up Against Sports Anxiety

As your athlete moves into more competitive levels, or if they begin to compete individually, it's normal to feel the presence of pregame jitters or nervousness. But if their pregame jitters make them weak or dizzy, or their nervousness turns into nausea, they may be experiencing sports anxiety.

Sports anxiety is a type of social anxiety that interferes with sports performance. Even the most elite athletes can suffer from high-stress situations resulting in loss of "muscle memory" and choking under pressure.

REMEMBER

Social anxiety disorder is a fear of being embarrassed or disappointing others, with a focus on how others will view a performance rather than the merits of the performance itself. For more on social anxiety see Chapter 4.

Looking for signs

In young children, the signs of sports anxiety are both within and outside of participation time. The following list includes the most common symptoms of sports anxiety:

>> Negative self-talk

>> Hesitation or decreased confidence during sport

>> Irritability or unusual behavior at home and on the field

>> Pretending to be sick or injured to avoid participation

>> Experiencing decreased levels of enjoyment or wanting to quit

Managing sports anxiety

The key principle for any athlete to learn is to focus on the things they can control and not waste energy on things they can't. The one thing your athlete can control is their own preparation, so that should be their full focus. The following are other suggestions that may help:

>> **Keep daily routines.** By developing consistent routines, uncertainty can be reduced, and your athlete is less likely to be negatively affected by external factors. This includes things like being on time to practice and games, keeping the sports bag ready and packed, and cleaning equipment in one consistent space so items don't get misplaced.

>> **Practice and teach calming techniques.** Self-regulation techniques like breath control and grounding (see Chapter 16), help reduce heart rate, relax muscles, and slow down breathing — all physical responses that impact athletic performance.

>> **Create preparatory routines (PRs).** PRs are predictable routines that take place directly before the start of an activity, like listening to the same playlist, running the same pregame drills, or putting on equipment in a routine fashion. PRs are learned and practiced in order to help athletes regulate their emotions, thoughts, behaviors, and performance.

>> **Prioritize sleep.** Sleep plays a major role in reaction time, coordination, energy levels, and anxiety management. Make sure your child gets plenty of sleep, especially in the days before an athletic event. For more on sleep see Chapter 13.

>> **Shift the focus.** Emphasize effort and goals related to teamwork. Have your basketball player focus on assists rather than points, and your volleyball player on digs rather than kills.

>> **Lean into professional help.** Your child may need professional help for sports anxiety if fear and stress interfere with their performance, well-being, or enjoyment. A sports therapist or sports psychologist can be a helpful way for your child to build coping strategies and restore confidence.

IN THIS CHAPTER

» Discovering how behaviors are
learned

» Evaluating elements of effective
behavior management

» Choosing and adapting behavior
management strategies for anxious
kids

» Handling challenging behavior

Chapter 15

Implementing Behavior Management Strategies

A large portion of your home's character is grounded in the parenting practices you choose to use. When you live with an anxious child, it's possible that changes to your behavior management strategies will help your home be more peaceful.

In this chapter, you find out how behaviors are learned and modified. In turn, you discover foundational components that should be present in any type of behavior management strategy you choose, as well as evidence-supported ways to change a child's behavior. Finally, you get a handle on elements of behavior management that are unique to a child with anxiety.

Understanding How Behaviors Are Learned

Children learn behaviors through a combination of observation, reinforcement, emotional adaptation, and repeated experiences. For example, a preschooler may learn to say "please" and "thank you" by watching their parents, receiving praise for using manners, noticing the positive response it brings, and repeating it during daily routines like meals or playdates.

Another key component of behavioral learning is emotional connection. When kids see their parents express fear, display confidence, or react to something new, they often imitate what they see. Additionally, secure relationships between parents and their children help kids develop emotional resilience.

One reason some behaviors stick and others fade away is reinforcement. Reinforcement comes in lots of forms. A familiar example is positive reinforcement, like receiving praise for completing homework or getting a sticker after a great checkup at the doctor's office. Related is negative reinforcement, or when the behavior removes a negative consequence. For kids with anxiety, this means avoidance.

WARNING

One of the hallmarks of anxiety disorders is *avoidance behavior* — escaping or avoiding situations that cause fear or discomfort. Just as rewards reinforce good behavior, avoidance reinforces irrational fears. By avoiding anxiety temporarily, the fear is strengthened over time. The problem with avoidance behaviors is that they prevent your child from understanding that a situation is safe or manageable, making future experiences even more distressing.

The following are some examples of common avoidance behaviors:

>> A second-grader takes an excessively long time to put on their soccer cleats before getting on the field, shortening their practice time.

>> A fourth-grader asks their parent to order for them at a restaurant, avoiding the need to talk to the waiter or make a decision under pressure.

>> A sixth-grader is worried about shots at the doctor's office, so they beg and plead with their parent to do it another day.

REMEMBER

Avoidance behaviors are part of your child's anxiety. Their brain is telling them to do these things to keep their body safe. To that end, no one should be punished or reprimanded for doing something that makes their body feel safe.

REMEMBER

Taking a confident and consistent role in your child's development is essential. You shape your child's behavior by providing structure, setting expectations, and responding to your child's actions with consistent consequences. Additionally, your interactions and decisions strengthen the bond with your child by fostering respect, emotional responsiveness, and love.

Recognizing a Positive Parenting Household

So, how can a child's behavior be successfully changed? Behavior management strategies help kids overcome their resistance, improve cooperation, and adopt better behavior. Effective approaches encourage good habits, redirect misbehavior, and build problem-solving skills. For kids with anxiety, behavior management includes being mindful of not reinforcing avoidance.

There are hundreds of ways to change a child's behavior, many of them defined as "right" or "wrong" by everyone from online influencers and celebrity parent experts to your own grandmother. Much of this advice is largely based on tradition and experience. To add clarity, psychological researchers have evaluated many techniques and found some to be more effective than others.

The most effective behavior management strategies used with young children include a blend of similar elements. Together, these form the characteristics of positive and relational parenting. The following sections look at some of these.

Building relationship

The human brain — yours and your child's — is structured to be in relationship with other people in a way that keeps them safe. You provide safety to your child in physical ways, like child-proofing your home, getting routine medical care, and taking them to school. Emotionally, you show safety with acceptance, encouragement, and love. Safety is also created by establishing boundaries and rules, and enforcing them consistently and calmly.

Effective behavior management techniques address the issue you're trying to improve, reinforce emotional and physical safety, and prioritize relationship at the same time. This requires a consistent and compassionate approach that redirects or removes undesired behaviors while instilling family values and showing respect.

Paying attention and empathizing

Empathy maintains relationships, even when correcting misbehavior. It involves understanding and reflecting your child's emotions, even if you don't agree with them. Nonverbal empathy includes nodding or mirroring expressions; verbal empathy involves describing feelings, asking questions, and validating emotions.

To empathize, you need to pay attention. You have to slow down, make eye contact, be aware of the context, ask questions, and be present. This directly competes with the distractions of modern life, like competing priorities, extra work, lack of sleep, mobile devices, and your own emotional well-being.

REMEMBER

You can empathize, even if you disagree. Showing understanding may help calm a child down and, when paired with a coping statement, can develop into effective self-talk that will regulate their own feelings (for example, "I see you are sad. Let's try something else instead.").

REMEMBER

It's impossible to be fully present every second. Plus, too much hovering leads to overprotective tendencies that inhibit your child's ability to develop autonomy and self-reliance. (For more about this anxiety-producing parenting style see Chapter 12.) But when you're inconsistently available, kids may feel ignored, rejected, or distressed, leading to more emotional outbursts. It's a balance.

Prioritizing safety

Behavior management must focus on keeping young kids safe. To do this, establishing boundaries is necessary. Of course, boundaries change as kids grow, from holding hands to cross a busy street to enforcing a teen's curfew. It's these types of boundaries that teach kids self-control, responsibility, and healthy decision-making.

Kids also require emotional safety. When they have strong emotions, they need to know that you'll be with them through the discomfort and feel welcomed back when they need to share with you again. This emotional safety is foundational for secure attachment that happens over time, decreasing anxiety and promoting emotional wellness over the relationship.

REMEMBER

Letting your child's anxiety control the household doesn't help anyone. Setting limits and learning strategies show kindness and care. Staying firm and consistent won't harm your child, but allowing a treatable problem to persist will.

Honoring developmental skills

Successful behavioral modification strategies need to be able to adapt to your child's developmental level. For preschoolers, redirection and consistent routines may be all that's needed for impulse control and reasoning skills. By school age, communication strategies and logical consequences better match their ability to understand cause and effect, regulate emotions, and take responsibility.

Promoting social-emotional learning

Being understood by an adult helps a child calm the powerful stress response so that their brain is in a calm and alert state for learning. When they are calm, kids can learn to identify, express, and manage their emotions in a healthy way rather than reacting impulsively.

TIP

Until your child is calm, they are unable to learn. Use the calming techniques (see Chapter 16) to get their thinking brain engaged before trying to explain or reason.

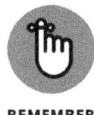

REMEMBER

During early childhood, emotions are stronger than cognitive skills. This natural imbalance, which I discuss in Chapter 2, is one reason why kids require behavior management. Until prefrontal cortex skills are increased, kids need constant reminders and direction in order to comprehend which behaviors align with your family goals and values. They can't do this on their own.

Creating and enforcing boundaries

Like bridge rails, household rules create safety and reduce anxiety by providing clear, reliable expectations. Modeling and coaching helps kids develop self-regulation, problem-solving, and relationship skills, and shape their moral responsibility and perspective-taking. Without limits, behavior lacks direction, leaving kids overwhelmed and more anxious. Boundaries make a safety zone where they can grow and explore with confidence.

The most effective boundaries tend to be created by you and your child together, giving your child some control within the safety of the boundaries you've set. When your child realizes that their input matters, they'll be more likely to adhere to the boundary. Of course, little kids need more direct guidance than older children.

REMEMBER

In the moment, it's okay (and expected) for your child to be unhappy when you enforce a boundary that has been set. It's part of a kid's DNA to test boundaries to ensure that *you* are following through. This is how they figure out how the world works, gain attention, assert independence, and express emotion. Approaching calmly and firmly, while being respectful, provides stability in this teaching.

REMEMBER

Enforcing boundaries won't jeopardize the connection with your child that you desire. Clear, fair limits provide a sense of security and show children that you're reliable and that rules exist for their well-being — not as a form of control or rejection.

Avoiding punishments and preparing consequences

To enforce boundaries, consequences are often needed. The essential piece is that the consequence must make sense. Here are a few examples:

>> If a child is ignoring directions, pause their activity (turn off the TV or the like) until they follow through with the request.

>> If a child is refusing to share, have them take a break from the item in question.

>> If a child is whining, let them know you're going to respond only when they use their regular voice.

TIP

Taking away screen time should be reserved for unwanted screen-related behaviors, like breaking the daily time limit, using the device in an unapproved location, or visiting websites they know are not approved for use. Randomly taking away screens for a variety of undesired behavior isn't effective; it increases your child's perceived value of screen time itself. This can make screen time battles much harder overall.

Consequence is different from punishment. A consequence is a logical or natural outcome of a behavior. In contrast, punishment prioritizes fear or discomfort, like extra chores, threats, or random removal of privileges. Children need problem-solving, not punishment. Clear boundaries and logical consequences are essential to this goal.

REMEMBER

Consequences teach; punishments control. If your response to an undesired behavior helps your child learn from their actions and make better choices next time, it's a logical consequence — if it only causes distress without teaching, it's a punishment.

Avoiding punishment is tough for every parent because punishment is *emotional.* Giving your child a punishment is an impulsive reaction when you're angry, embarrassed, or frustrated. And although a punishment may get a reaction in the short term, it's not helping you accomplish the goal. Consequences take a bit of planning and preparation, but they have more long-term effectiveness to create the behavior patterns you would like to see in your child.

WARNING

Extensive psychological and neurobiological research has shown significant negative effects when using any form of corporal punishment in young children. There is *never* a justification or reason to hit a child. Kids don't have to "learn their lesson" or suffer in some way in order to create behavior change.

Using clear communication

Clear communication ensures that your child understands expectations, consequences, and the reasons behind rules. When you use simple, direct, and consistent language, your kids are more likely to follow rules and learn from mistakes. Clear communication also reduces frustration, builds trust, and encourages cooperation, helping what you're asking to feel fair rather than punitive.

TIP

For young kids, clear communication often includes breaking big tasks into smaller steps. Communicating each step individually will increase success. For example, instead of telling your child to get ready for bed, tell them to put on their pajamas, brush their teeth, and pick out a book. Or, more simply, "It's PJs, brush, and book time!"

Prioritizing space for self-care

Stressed, overworked, and frustrated parents are ineffective. Space for parental self-care allows you to maintain patience and stay emotionally balanced. When you are well-rested and emotionally regulated, you're better able to respond calmly and thoughtfully to misbehavior, rather than react impulsively. This naturally creates a stable environment where your child is more likely to thrive and learn.

Choosing Effective Strategies

Children with anxiety respond to certain behavioral strategies better than others. This often requires knowledge of a few different types of strategies to adapt your response to the situation or type of misbehavior. Specific details and descriptions of each type of behavioral management technique is outside the scope of this book. However, you'll find elements of the positive practices from the last section in each of the following recommended techniques:

>> **Positive reinforcement:** Use rewards to encourage behaviors you want to see more of. This can mean earning a sticker for getting ready for school without reminders. The key is to reinforce the behavior right after it happens.

>> **Pre-correction and prompting:** Anticipate moments of stress — like transitions or undesired tasks — and set them up for success with verbal cues or instructions. For example, before leaving the playground say, "In five minutes, we're heading to the car. I will need calm walking and listening ears."

>> **Attention to desired behavior:** Reinforce the positive or "catch them being good." Notice and praise small efforts toward positive behaviors to help them know what to repeat, like saying, "I saw you take a deep breath instead of yelling — great job calming down."

>> **Planned ignoring:** Intentionally withhold your attention from undesired behaviors. Use this for minor attention-seeking behaviors like whining or interrupting. As soon as the behavior stops, shift your attention back with engagement.

>> **Behavior contract:** Provide clear behavior expectations in writing. Work together on a list of specific behaviors and rewards or consequences. Post the contract in a visible place and review it regularly.

>> **Active listening and problem-solving:** Understand the situation first, then guide next steps. Use phrases like "It sounds like you were frustrated when that happened." Once they feel heard, help them brainstorm better responses for the next time.

>> **Natural and logical consequences:** Offer real-world outcomes that relate directly to the behavior. If a toy is thrown, it's removed for the day. This helps kids see the impact of their choices and learn from them.

TIP

For any behavioral management strategy you choose, use the following questions as a checklist to ensure that you are headed in the right direction:

>> Does this strategy help my child grow and develop a life skill?

>> Is this building our relationship or harming it?

>> Is this developmentally appropriate?

>> Is this strategy consistent and predictable, yet flexible to the situation?

>> Would I want this done to me?

Tailoring Strategies for Kids with Anxiety

Anxiety comes from fear. Fear leads to irrational and unwanted behaviors. When redirecting misbehaviors in anxious kids, there are a few things to keep in mind with the strategy you choose.

Searching for context

Your child's behaviors may be directly driven by their irrational fear and not something they can easily control. Initially, this can be hard to see. It often takes awareness of your child's anxiety triggers and some time to find these patterns. The following are a couple of examples.

REMEMBER

You can't take anxiety away from your child, but you can create an environment that reinforces healthy behaviors and helps them manage it on their own.

Displaying defiance

Here is Angela's story:

> Angela is a 5-year-old who is becoming restless in the evenings. She refuses to put on her pajamas, asks for multiple snacks, insists she needs another story, and keeps coming out of her room. Her parents grow frustrated, assuming she's just being defiant and trying to manipulate them into staying up later. As a consequence, they try taking away stories, making the behavior worse.

Angela is showing signs of separation anxiety, not defiance. She's using tactics to keep parents close so she doesn't feel scared. Once her parents discovered her anxiety, they changed their strategy to offering comfort, creating a consistent bedtime routine that included breathing technique practice, and began a plan to gradually shorten the time they would stay in her room. After a few weeks, the tantrums stopped and the bedtime routine was enjoyable again.

Harrowing homework

Here is Amy's story:

> Amy is a 9-year-old who is sitting at the kitchen table, staring at a math worksheet with tears in her eyes. She tells her mom, "I can't do this. It's too hard." Her mother, chopping vegetables at the kitchen sink, says, "If you just focused instead of crying about it, you'd be done by now. Finish it up so you can go play." This makes Amy cry harder and she slams her pencil on the table, breaking it into bits.

Amy isn't trying to avoid her homework — she's experiencing anxiety with perfectionism. She believes that if she can't get the answer right immediately, she has failed. Her anxious brain tells her that making mistakes is unacceptable, so instead of working through the problem, she freezes or panics.

After a few nights of this repeated behavior, her mom changed her approach. She validated Amy's frustration, helped her break the assignment into smaller sections, and praised her effort to try one more section on her own. Over time, math homework was getting done more quickly and without the tears.

Creating consistency

Consistency eases anxiety. Predictable environments help anxious kids, which is why routines (see Chapter 13) are effective. Consistency in behavior management includes having intentional conversations — when your child is calm — about your family rules, expectations, and consequences.

Explain to your child what you're doing and why. If your child misbehaves, remind them about the rules when you give the consequence. If you need a new rule based on new behavior, state it clearly. Then, stick to it — knowing what to expect reduces anxiety.

TIP

One tool to create consistency is using a *behavioral contract.* This is a written agreement between you and your child that outlines expected behaviors, rewards for meeting expectations, and consequences for not following through. Contracts are often more effective for anxious kids than relying exclusively on natural consequences, which are too variable.

Clarifying "zero tolerance"

Some actions aren't tolerated under any circumstances, even when a child is anxious. For most families, these actions include things like swearing, hitting, stealing, damaging property, deliberately harming others or pets, and verbal assaults.

Clearly define your "zero tolerance" behaviors and consequences with your child. Immediately take action if those are violated. Hold your anxious child to the same behavior standards as others.

TIP

Anxious kids tend to be perfectionistic. Be clear that it's their behavior that you are not happy with, not them as a person. Use words that reflect this distinction. For example, "That doesn't feel like you. Can we talk about what's going on?" Or, to affirm effort, say, "I see how hard you tried. One rough moment doesn't undo that."

Calming first

When anxious kids get overwhelmed and are unable to avoid something, or you don't let them, they will go into a more extreme stress reaction. When this happens, anxious kids will fight, scream, run, and yell.

Be ready for your child's reaction and have a plan. Your job in these moments is to de-escalate. You need to get them to a safe place, co-regulate, validate, and remain calm. When you take the bait, escalate, or punish this behavior, the anxiety wins.

It's only when your child has calmed down that their thinking brain will re-engage, allowing them to more rationally think about the initial trigger and their response. You will get more information when your child is calm. What set them off? Why did they get so upset? What else could they have done at that moment?

After gathering information, then you can remind them about your family's rules and discuss a consequence, if needed. Whatever you choose should be related to behavior and encourage them to make better choices in the future.

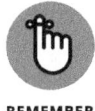

REMEMBER

It can be maddening when your 6-year-old can clearly state a family rule when they are calm, only to do the opposite when they are emotionally overwhelmed. Be patient and don't lose faith in the process. Your consistent response will be effective over time.

Modeling imperfection

Modeling your own imperfections teaches your child that mistakes are normal and not something to fear. When children see you handle setbacks with patience and problem-solving, they learn to do the same.

For example, if you burn dinner, instead of getting frustrated, you can say, "Oops, I messed up the recipe. No big deal — I'll try again or make something else." This shows your child that mistakes aren't failures but opportunities to learn.

By openly acknowledging imperfections and handling them with resilience, you help your child see that they don't need to be perfect to be successful or valued. Over time, this reduces their anxiety about making mistakes and encourages a healthier, more flexible mindset.

Avoiding avoidance

When your child feels anxious, their brain reacts as if there is a real danger, even when there isn't. This leads them to avoid situations, shut down, or react in ways that actually make their anxiety worse. As a parent, you may need to gently guide them toward doing the *opposite* of what their anxious brain is telling them to do.

Simply forcing your child to step into situations without tools to manage anxious thoughts and physical sensations won't work in the long term. The goal is to help your child learn how to tolerate uncertainty, be flexible, walk through uncomfortable sensations, and manage their behavior.

TIP

For kids who need constant reassurance, it's okay to ignore the repeated questions. Instead, tell your child that when they ask about [insert repeat topic here], you're going to ignore the question and reply with a random code word like "maracas." Then, when your child repeatedly asks something you know is fueled by anxiety, simply reply, "I hear you. Maracas." Then move on to something else.

Catching your child being brave

When a child receives praise or comfort for avoiding a feared situation, avoidance is reinforced. Conversely, if bravery is encouraged and rewarded, they are more likely to repeat the brave behavior.

If you choose to use rewards, give them for accomplishments that are important, difficult, or uncomfortable, or that require significant effort. Being brave as an anxious kid is hard work; reward the effort and willingness to try a small step.

TIP

Select rewards that you feel comfortable giving and that are convenient and readily available. Depending on your child's age and interests, some options will be better than others. The following are some options:

>> Getting a night off from doing chores

>> Having a friend over

>> Eating at a restaurant of their choice on a family night out

>> Choosing the movie on movie night

>> Getting rewards such as pencils, stickers, or craft supplies; hair accessories; or action figures

Again, rewards should be for big, hard things. After a reward is earned, give it as soon as you can. Then, talk with your child about the next thing you're watching for in order to earn the next reward, appropriately stretching their comfort zone and challenging them to try new things.

Managing Challenging Behavior

It's normal for kids to push boundaries and take risks. If your child has anxiety, their pushback can escalate so quickly that it becomes very difficult to positively intervene. If you feel yourself being challenged by your child's behavior, here are a few things to consider:

>> **Make sure your expectations are age appropriate.** Your anxious child likely already has high expectations for themselves, so be mindful of setting expectations too high or too low. Overestimating their abilities adds stress as they push to please you.

REMEMBER

Underestimating your child weakens their confidence. When you believe they can, they'll find it easier to believe it too.

>> **Try to keep your own emotions in check, including any anxiety you may feel.** Getting upset or angry can make

your child's anxiety worse. It may also make it harder for your child to take in and remember what you're saying.

Yelling is not a skill. It's an emotional reaction.

>> **Beware the anxious tantrum.** When you accommodate anxious tantruming, the anxiety and its controlling behaviors will get stronger — and it will happen quickly.

>> **Work with one strategy for a while.** Don't change strategies too soon. It can take a few weeks to begin to see effectiveness. Also, quick changes in expectations will make kids more anxious. Give you and your child time to see whether a strategy is working. If a plan needs to change, clearly and calmly communicate the new expectations.

>> **Be prepared to be consistent.** Giving in sometimes — intermittently reinforcing a behavior — makes a behavior much stronger, like a slot machine payout. If a child learns a behavior that works to get what they want, especially occasionally, they become obsessed with it.

Kids don't need perfect parents; they need predictable parents.

>> **Consider co-morbidity.** Anxiety may not be the only thing that is making your child's behaviors challenging. Talk to your child's care provider if you are concerned.

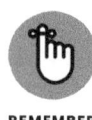

>> **Recognize that sometimes you just don't know the answer to challenging behavior.** Some of you are naturally great at building emotional connections but find enforcing boundaries and consequences very difficult. Others of you can guide behavior easily with consequences but struggle to keep your connection strong while doing so. Finding the middle ground is hard for all of us, which is why there is help. There are therapists and counselors trained in behavior management strategies who may be able to offer help for your specific challenges.

Chapter **16**

Calming Techniques and Why They Work

Young children navigate life using instinctive, emotion-driven reactions, all aimed at self-preservation. Watch a group of preschoolers at snack time, and you'll see what I mean. As kids' brains develop and they gain life experience, they gradually shift from reacting impulsively to emotions, to managing and expressing them with more control. Until this transition happens, children need caregivers to help guide them toward self-regulation.

In this chapter, you find out how children develop the self-regulation skills required to manage their emotions, and why these skills are essential for lifelong mental wellness. I introduce calming techniques to help build self-regulation and show you how to teach and use these skills with your child as they grow. Lastly, I cover panic attacks in kids, including how to recognize them and how to support a child through an attack.

Calming the Brain and Body

Regulation is the ability to manage emotions and behavior in response to changing circumstances. Early on, children rely on caregivers for this guidance, but as they grow, they develop *self-regulation* (SR) — the ability to calm and control automatic reactions on their own. SR is a complex skill that depends on brain development, life experiences, executive functioning, temperament, and memory.

SR plays a crucial role in shaping a child's mental health and well-being. It fosters healthy relationships, aids learning, and builds resilience. Research shows that strong SR skills strongly predict academic success, career achievement, and overall health; weak SR skills increase risks of peer conflicts and academic struggles. Children with poor SR are also more prone to anxiety.

Managing anxiety with self-regulation

Anxiety, fear, and worry can trigger a surge of stress hormones that powerfully activate the emotional brain, functionally disconnecting it from the thinking brain. When this happens, kids' ability to use logic and reason is drastically limited. In other words, when stress gets high, a child's thinking brain goes "offline," making it difficult for them to think clearly. SR skills keep a child's thinking brain "online" during emotional moments. But to be effective tools, these skills must be taught and consistently practiced.

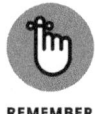

REMEMBER

No matter what a child's IQ or perceived maturity is, they cannot fully self-regulate until certain brain areas develop. So, don't get frustrated when they lose emotional control — it's normal! They need your guidance to build these skills as they grow.

SR develops gradually and hierarchically, much like the other milestones I describe in Chapter 2. Early SR skills lay the foundation for more advanced skills, which become increasingly complex and effective over time. An early SR skill in a 5-year-old may be managing frustration when losing a board game. A 10-year-old demonstrates SR by stepping away from a tough math problem without giving up. By adolescence and adulthood, SR evolves to include goal-setting, complex problem-solving, time management, and conflict resolution.

Building self-regulation skills

Children learn SR skills in a variety of ways. They develop SR by interacting with friends, navigating social dynamics, managing wins and losses, and resolving conflicts. In addition, many of your daily parenting activities support SR growth. Activities like imaginative play, board games, and storytelling, as well as creating predictable routines and safe spaces to manage emotions at home, all help SR grow.

SR skills can also be directly taught by equipping kids with tools to navigate future challenges. One powerful way to teach SR is through calming techniques. These strategies help children recognize and manage their emotional and physical responses to stress.

Calming techniques help reduce anxiety symptoms and impulsivity while building emotional, cognitive, and behavioral self-control. They teach kids to pause and manage stress on their own, while also strengthening their emotional connection with you. With practice, they become lifelong skills for mental well-being.

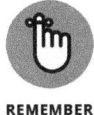

REMEMBER

Emotions are innate; SR skills are not. Strengthening these skills helps kids manage anxiety in the moment, while laying the foundation for lifelong mental and physical well-being.

Teaching Calming Techniques to Your Child

Have you ever told a tantruming child, "You need to calm down"? An angry middle schooler to "get over it"? How did that turn out? I'm guessing not well.

Using trite phrases during stressful moments with kids (and other adults) only amplifies frustration while limiting opportunity for constructive support. I challenge you to break this habit and practice calming techniques to help both you and your child during the next emotional moment, building SR along the way. Kids as young as age 3 can use these techniques, but they can't do it alone. Learning SR requires great coaching, age-appropriate expectations, and plenty of patience. *You* are just the person they need! The following are five essential parts to teaching any calming technique.

Timing matters

You can't teach calming techniques in the heat of the moment. The thinking brain is "offline" during stress, and limited learning can take place. Instead, teach these techniques when your child is calm, allowing for low-stakes practice in a positive setting.

TIP

Building calming practice into your daily routine removes any awkwardness and builds a great habit. Bedtime is an ideal time, or consider the car ride to school or sports practice as other routine opportunities.

Learning together

Find a few calming techniques your child enjoys and can reliably use. Explore different options and practice together; you'll find examples later in this chapter. For older kids, explaining why and how these techniques work can increase their buy-in. Keep in mind that these techniques are beneficial for you, too!

Using co-regulation

Until your child develops complex SR skills, you can help them learn though *co-regulation.* During co-regulation, you intentionally cooperate with your child by sharing your thinking patterns and behaviors to demonstrate SR skills. Your child can then mimic these strategies and gradually use them independently.

Successful co-regulation doesn't remove the stressor. Instead, it empowers your child to work through anxiety on their own. Be mindful to avoid accommodation behaviors (see Chapter 12) you use when your child is stressed — they derail the SR learning process.

Trusting the process

Like any learning journey, using calming techniques has ups and downs. It takes practice to spot the early signs of anxiety and apply techniques before things get overwhelming. With consistent use over time, you'll notice your child responding more quickly to your cues, reducing the duration and frequency of dysregulated moments.

It's wildly frustrating when your child can explain how to breathe and calm their body . . . after having a 15-minute meltdown. During a tantrum, their thinking brain is "offline," making it hard to remember and use calming techniques. Practice together, and be patient.

Exploring Calming Techniques

There are hundreds of calming techniques to manage stress, but no single strategy works for every person or situation. It's important to have a large toolbox of techniques. This section includes a few of my favorite breath control, grounding, and cognitive engagement techniques to get you started.

Start by teaching and practicing breath control. It's one of the quickest ways to de-escalate stress.

Breath control

There are innumerable types of breathing techniques, all serving the same physiological purpose. Deep breathing activates your parasympathetic nervous system and vagus nerve, helping your body chill out by slowing your heart rate, lowering blood pressure, and conserving energy. By breathing deeply and slowly, you can control the stressful experience.

One example of breath control is *box breathing*. Practice the following steps with your child to use this technique:

1. **Visualize a box with four equal sides.**

Each side represents a phase of your breath.

2. **Breathe in through your nose for a count of 4.**

Imagine you're drawing the first side of the box.

3. **Hold your breath for a count of 4, visualizing the next side.**

4. **Breathe out through your mouth for a count of 4.**

Empty your lungs, drawing the third side of the box in your mind.

5. **Hold your breath for a count of 4.**

Complete the box by imagining the fourth side.

Repeat box breathing until your child feels relaxed and calm. Adjust the length of each side of the box as needed for your child, such as two or three seconds per side, keeping each side consistent. While practicing, have your child "draw" a box in their palm to help their focus. Teach them to move air by moving their belly in and out, not lifting their shoulders up and down.

Alternatively, teach deep, slow breathing by pretending to blow out candles or blow down a building. Props like soap bubbles or pinwheels can encourage strong exhalations. Humming or singing while slowing breathing will also stimulate the vagus nerve.

TIP

Many people believe the depth of the breath triggers calm, but it's the *exhalation* that activates the parasympathetic effect. Make sure your child is moving their belly to fully exhale during any breathing practice.

Grounding

Grounding techniques help a person focus on the present moment through sensory awareness. They interrupt the stress response by redirecting feelings of stress, while engaging the parasympathetic nervous system and thinking brain.

Focusing on the five senses

One commonly used grounding technique is called the 5-4-3-2-1 exercise. During this practice, you walk through the five senses. Take a deep belly breath to begin, then slowly work through the following steps:

1. **Look for five things you can see, saying the objects out loud.**

   For example, you can say, "I see the computer, I see the mug, I see the door, I see the window, I see the phone."

2. **Name four things you can feel, and say them out loud.**

   For example, say, "I feel my warm feet in my socks, the chair that I'm sitting on, the book that I'm holding, and the mug of hot tea."

3. **Listen for three sounds.**

   Call out the sounds of the birds outside, the traffic passing by, or the radio playing.

4. **Say two things you can smell.**

   If you can't smell anything, name two favorite smells.

5. **Say one thing you can taste.**

   Maybe the toothpaste from brushing your teeth or the taste of your gum. If you aren't tasting anything, name a favorite flavor. Take a deep belly breath to end the practice.

Alternatively, you can try the 3-3-3 exercise by modifying the preceding list to three things you see, hear, and smell.

TIP

If sensations are too difficult, ask your child to name something in their environment according to the letters of the alphabet. Start by asking your child to find something that starts with A, then B, then C, and so forth. Let them go through as many letters as they can before checking in with how they feel.

Grounding exercises can also use direct sensory stimulation to interrupt stress signals, reducing the intensity and duration of the stress response. The following list offers examples of how to engage your child's senses:

>> Give them a sour candy or strongly flavored gum to chew.

>> Have them hold an ice cube or place their hands in icy water.

>> Clap a pattern and have them repeat it.

>> Imitate an animal noise, and have them guess the animal and repeat it.

>> Let them squeeze a stress ball or play with scented Play-Doh.

Making the most of movement

TIP

Movement is also grounding, and kids love to move! It reduces stress hormones and gives the brain physical input to disrupt the stress response. The following are examples of movement techniques:

>> Wall push-ups or arm circles

>> Jumping jacks, dance moves, or jumping rope

>> Rocking or swinging

>> Self-hug or bear hugs

>> Balancing on one foot or walking along a straight line

Cognitive engagement

Cognitive techniques engage the thinking brain, keeping it "online" to help with emotional interpretation and feedback. These techniques strengthen the prefrontal cortex and promote neurotransmitter balance. They also interrupt negative feedback loops to challenge unhelpful thoughts and encourage relaxation.

Cognitively engage your child by having them count as high as they can by fives, or having them count backwards from 100 by sixes. Alternatively, they can think of a food or animal for each letter of the alphabet (for example, A is for apple, B is for banana). Playing I Spy or 20 Questions is also an effective go-to. All these cognitive techniques engage the prefrontal cortex, support rational thinking and emotional regulation, and help your anxious child calm down.

Putting Calming Techniques into Action

No matter the calming technique you use, using them within a consistent framework of support will help your child anticipate and apply the tool. The following list describes your action steps:

>> **Label the emotion.** Identifying and naming your child's emotions is an essential part of emotional development and SR. By observing their behavior or listening to what they express, calmly name the emotion you think they're experiencing, even if you're unsure. Naming emotions helps build their emotional vocabulary, normalizes their emotional experiences, and strengthens your parent-child bond.

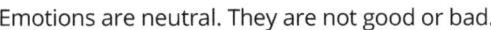

Emotions are neutral. They are not good or bad.

REMEMBER

>> **Stick to the basics.** Avoid complicating the emotional label with projections or moral judgments. For example, a 4-year-old who just hit their brother likely feels anger, not remorse or regret — those are more complex emotions. Keeping it simple and honest is key.

Psychology experts commonly agree that the basic human emotions are fear, anger, joy, sadness, disgust, and surprise.

TECHNICAL
STUFF

>> **Validate their feelings.** During emotional moments, kids want to feel seen and heard. Validation is a communication technique you can use to show your child that it's okay to feel the way they do. Validation is a calm, empathetic, and nonjudgmental statement that reflects what your child's words or behaviors are expressing. Validation does not mean that you agree with their behavior or imply that their feelings are correct. It's simply a statement meant to foster

trust and support, allowing solution-focused communication to follow. The following are some examples:

- "It sounds like you are angry. We can come back to the park another day."
- "I took the iPad away, and I see you are mad."
- "It looks like you are scared. It's okay to feel scared, but nothing is going to hurt you."

Feelings are the interpretations of emotions, which may or may not be true.

≫ **Choose and co-regulate.** Quickly scan the situation and choose a technique that is familiar and accessible to your child. Cue your child to start using the technique verbally or with a "secret sign," like a tug on the ear or pat on the back. If needed, co-regulate by starting the technique and giving your child space to join in.

≫ **Attend to the desired behavior.** Be ready to offer encouragement for any SR attempts. Give positive attention for any behavior you want to encourage, even if your child is still upset. For example, praise your child for trying to take belly breaths, even though they're still sobbing. Catch the small moments of calm or cooperation to encourage positive behavior. If needed, follow through with a consequence to undesired behavior using an effective behavior management technique *after the event is over*. You can find out more in Chapter 15.

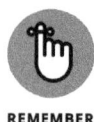

All emotions are welcome, but all behaviors are not.

≫ **Model consistently.** Between stressful episodes, model this process in your own day. Articulate your emotions and how you use SR techniques. Though it may feel awkward, there's power in *showing*. Your children are always watching, and when you show them your process, you have the power to normalize and teach SR skills they can use in the future.

Being a great parent doesn't mean your child is always happy — that would be unrealistic. The goal is to raise a young adult who is able to manage what life throws at them using effective SR practices. Achieving this through a positive relationship full of collaboration and love — that's great parenting.

Dealing with Panic Attacks in Kids

A panic attack is a sudden, intense event that triggers a dramatic cascade of emotional and physical responses. Recognizing what a panic attack looks like in kids is important to understand anxiety's various forms. However, I discuss these separately from anxiety and calming techniques for two reasons:

>> Panic attacks are uncommon in young children.

>> Panic attacks require unique support from caregivers, unlike normal tantrums or outbursts.

Dissecting what happens to the body during a panic attack

Panic attacks start when the *amygdala*, a key region of the emotional brain that processes fear, activates a cascade of hormones and neurotransmitters that affect nearly every body system — imagine a "flight-or-fight" reaction happening without warning. The attack continues until the natural chemicals triggering the reaction slowly dissolve into nonfunctional fragments. In other words, once this powerful fear cascade begins, the effects cannot be immediately stopped. A person experiencing a panic attack can only ride down the symptoms until these hormones and neurotransmitters have dispersed.

TECHNICAL
STUFF

Many symptoms of a panic attack are from a surge of epinephrine and norepinephrine. The sudden and dramatic rise of these neurotransmitters creates a physiological imbalance, leaving relative low levels of calming neurotransmitters, like serotonin and GABA, available to dampen the fear response.

Panic attacks are frightful for both the child experiencing the attack and those around them. Especially in young children, the chest tightness, difficulty breathing, trembling, or abdominal discomfort can be so severe that parents take their child to the emergency room for help. In fact, kids are often seen in medical facilities to confirm that the symptoms are due to panic and not another medical condition.

Identifying panic

All panic attacks have a constellation of physical and emotional symptoms, although the presentation may be different for each attack. Find out more through the experience of Stephanie, a 10-year-old girl who recently moved to a new school:

> At 8:30 p.m., Stephanie begins her usual bedtime routine. As bedtime approaches, she becomes more agitated.
>
> By 8:45 p.m., she refuses to go to bed, pacing and crying uncontrollably. Her breathing becomes rapid, and she complains of feeling "hot and sweaty," with tingling in her hands and feet. She curls up, trembling, saying she's "too scared to sleep" and can't stop thinking something bad will happen at school the next day. When her parents try to console her, she pulls away and rushes to the bathroom, insisting she's going to throw up.
>
> Initially, her parents try reasoning with her, saying, "You're fine. There's nothing to worry about," but it only upsets her more. Her father sits beside her, speaks calmly, and encourages her to slow her breathing. After struggling to follow along, Stephanie starts to mimic him, and her breathing gradually slows. By 9:10 p.m., she's calmer, apologizes, and says, "I don't know why this happens." Her parents reassure her, promise to help her understand, and spend a few minutes reading a calming book before she settles into bed.

In this scenario, Stephanie is having a panic attack. Her symptoms are intense, sudden, and escalate to a level that is hard for her to control. Her attack requires unique support from her family to manage her emotional and physical symptoms. These characteristics differentiate Stephanie's panic episode from more commonly experienced anxiety attacks. For a more detailed comparison, see Table 16-1.

TABLE 16-1

Characteristics of Panic and Anxiety Attacks in Children

Feature	Panic Attack	Anxiety Attack
Onset	Sudden, without warning. Rare in younger children, more common in kids 10 and older.	Gradual, triggered by a stressor (a test, separation from family, social situation). Can begin as early as preschool age.
Duration	Brief, peaks in 10–15 minutes and resolves within 30–60 minutes.	Can last for hours or longer, or persist as chronic anxiety until stressor is resolved.
Physical symptoms	Severe: rapid heart rate, chest pain, nausea and vomiting, trembling, pins and needles sensation, feeling detached from reality.	Mild to moderate: tension, nausea, headache, or breathing changes. Much less intense than in panic.
Emotional symptoms	Overwhelming fear, sense of doom.	Persisting worry or dread, restlessness, preoccupation with feared event.
Frequency	Occasional and random, unless recurrent in panic disorder.	Linked to a specific event or stressor.

Appreciating panic's uniqueness

Unlike anxiety attacks, panic attacks have a few interesting features that make their treatment and management distinctive. The following list offers details:

>> **Panic attacks occur without warning.** The when, why, and how of panic attacks are unpredictable, and it's the sudden escalation of symptoms that makes SR techniques less effective. However, recognizing the early signs of an attack and actively working to suppress it can help limit the intensity and duration. Achieving this often requires professional support.

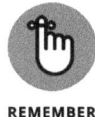

A predictable emotional and physical response to a known stressor or trigger is characteristic of an anxiety disorder. It's the extreme symptoms without a known trigger that make panic attacks unique.

>> **Panic attacks aren't limited to panic disorder.** A single panic attack doesn't mean your child has panic disorder. Panic

disorder is characterized by recurrent, unexpected attacks that cause persistent worry about their recurrence. For more about the diagnosis of panic disorder see Chapter 4.

>> **Panic attacks can be triggered by substances.** Caffeine, alcohol, and certain medications can stimulate stress hormones and trigger a panic cascade. In addition, certain sounds or smells that remind you of a stressful event can trigger panic symptoms. Although these triggers differ from amygdala-induced responses, the sequence of hormone and neurotransmitter release is fairly universal.

WARNING

Energy drinks and energy shots are known to cause panic attacks. Products with excessively high levels of caffeine are not recommended for kids.

>> **Panic attacks can be triggered by medical conditions.** Commonly experienced medical conditions like asthma, headaches, and allergic reactions can cause significant body stress and trigger the panic cascade.

>> **Panic attacks can cause a "hangover."** The surge of hormones and neurotransmitters during a panic attack is so strong that the body needs to recover. After an attack, it's not uncommon for your child to experience fatigue, irritability, dizziness, muscle tension, or a heightened sense of anxiety. These symptoms can be improved with hydration, rest, and light physical activity.

Supporting your child during a panic attack

When your child is having a panic attack, your support needs to align with what's happening in their brain and body. The fear response has essentially shut down your child's thinking brain, so *you* become the source of rational thinking and emotional regulation. Your goals are to capture your child's attention, co-regulate with them, and ride down the panic cascade together.

REMEMBER

In times of stress or panic, your role is not to identify the cause or fix the problem. Instead, offer compassion and support until the event passes. Understanding and problem-solving can come later.

If your child is having a panic attack, follow these supportive steps:

1. **Stay calm.**

   Though it's easier said than done, staying calm is critical! During fear or stress, your child looks to you for how to respond. Any anxiety or fear you show can confirm their behavior, potentially amplifying the panic response. Even if you're panicking on the inside, do your best to show calm in your face, body, and voice.

2. **Ensure their safety.**

   Do a quick scan of the area for any dangerous objects, places, or situations that need to be removed.

3. **Label and reassure.**

   Use short sentences and clear words. Tell your child they are having a panic attack, it will pass in a few minutes, and they are safe. Help them get through the peak by saying something like the following:

   - "I know you don't feel okay, but this will not hurt you. I will help you through this. It will end soon."

   - "These symptoms are scary, but your body is safe. I am not leaving. This feeling will end soon."

   - "This is a panic attack. It's harmless and nothing is wrong with your body. Keep thinking calmly, and this will pass."

   The panic cascade is physiologically consistent and predictable. Most panic attacks peak in about 10 minutes and resolve in 15–30 minutes.

4. **Control breathing.**

   With a reassuring presence, begin exaggerated and quiet belly breathing that your child can see, and ask them to join in when they are ready. During panic, this type of co-regulation is essential; you must actively and intentionally provide support. Limit talking, but it's okay to ask whether they need anything. If physical touch is desired, use firm and consistent pressure.

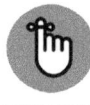

Control your breath; control your brain. By controlling your breathing, you take control of the panic response.

5. **Begin a grounding technique.**

Stay with your child and keep breathing. Once they begin to follow along, begin one of the grounding techniques they have practiced.

6. **Regroup.**

After the panic attack has passed, continue your reassurance and support. Give them a few moments to recover on their own. Once an appropriate amount of time has passed, hours to days, go back to the situation and see what they remember.

TIP

Keep a diary of your child's panic attacks, noting the timing, duration, and any context clues. Track which breathing and grounding techniques were most effective in helping them recover. Although the specifics may change, this record can be valuable to share with a professional or another caregiver if needed.

Chapter **17**

Focusing on Specific Concerns and Worries

I t's impossible to address all the infinite complexities that families of children with anxiety experience. However, throughout my years of clinical experience, I've noticed a few common situations that may apply to you. If that's the case, this chapter is someplace to get you started.

In this chapter, you find out how to get your anxious child to sleep, including techniques to stop bedsharing and details on sleep supplements. You also discover why toddlers and preteens are more prone to anxiety and when to reach out for help. Finally, you find a few things to consider when co-parenting an anxious child.

Getting an Anxious Child to Sleep

Children with anxiety often have sleep disruptions and resist bedtime. In Chapter 13 I explain how repeated anxious nights can cause negative associations with bedtime, leading to an increased reliance on parental involvement to fall asleep and reactive bedsharing.

Working toward better nighttime routines and increasing a child's sleep independence is possible, but it's not easy. There are no quick fixes. Re-associating your child's bedtime with calm, quiet, and comfort requires deliberate sleep training steps.

Sleep training is notoriously difficult for parents, and understandably so. Making changes that may *increase* your child's perceived bedtime stress may seem counterintuitive, unsupportive, even mean. Some parents simply cannot endure a child's crying without tremendous feelings of guilt or distress, or have cultural or physical considerations that make sleep training undesirable. And misinformation about the goal and consequences of the sleep training process remain a roadblock for many.

In my opinion, routine healthy sleep for the family is vital to protect from anxiety's harms. In turn, any benefits of evidence-supported sleep training far outweigh the perceived short-term distress that training may cause. All effective and safe training methods involve setting firm parental boundaries and teaching your child not to be fearful of their own bed, and also removing anxiety-driven sleep associations in supportive, structured, and sustainable ways.

REMEMBER

If you're happy with how your family is sleeping and everyone is getting great rest, sleep training isn't required. These methods are included here to help families who want to make changes to their child's bedtime experience.

The following techniques are evidence-based approaches to help children regain confidence in independent sleep. When done correctly, these will safely correct sleeping issues in over 80 percent of anxious kids. For most of my families who lead their child through this process, their experience is not full of regret or distress. Rather, they say, "I should have done that months ago."

TIP

Start with the good bedtime habits that I describe in Chapter 13. Have a plan with a firm start date with no upcoming vacations, transitions, or visitors. Training may be more efficient outside of the cold and flu season, since illnesses can derail progress.

TIP

For most of these methods, you should start seeing results in 2–3 weeks. If you aren't seeing any progress, talk with your doctor or therapist about alternative plans or sleep-focused cognitive behavioral therapy. For a child with extreme nighttime anxiety, medications can be tools to make the work of retraining easier on the parent and child. For more about medication see Chapter 10.

The Yale Program

Described by Dr. Eli Leibowitz, a child and adolescent psychologist at Yale University, this training method extinguishes reactive bedsharing by turning bedtime into a game. To use, describe to your child that staying in bed is part of a show, and they are the main character. Their job is to "trick" the audience into thinking they are going to sleep in their own bed, but they really aren't.

During bedtime, complete your normal routine, and then it's time for the show! Tell your child to get into bed and "fool" the audience by pretending to sleep. Be clear that the show is only a certain length of time — as little as 1 minute in length. After the show is over, you go into their room and get them — even if they appear comfortable — welcoming them back into your bed for the rest of the night. Increase the length of the "show" by a few minutes over a few nights, building up to 15–20 consecutive minutes. At that point, most kids fall asleep on their own.

The Yale Program works by re-associating time in bed with calm, using an expected time limit. Since kids know the time in bed is only for a short period, they don't ramp up their stress sequence. Instead, they work on building a new association of being relaxed in bed. For more details about the Yale Program see the Appendix.

The bedtime pass

The bedtime pass technique helps keep your child in their own bed by putting them in charge of their bedtime experience, while you remain in control. To use this technique, give your child a number of predetermined bedtime passes as you tuck them into their bed (for example, an index card or sticker). After lights-out, each pass can be exchanged by your child to get out of bed for a hug, drink of water, or brief reassurance. The pass is then returned to you and cannot be reused. For any passes not used in the morning, they can earn a small reward. Decrease the number of available passes over time.

TIP

Words matter. During the bedtime routine, focus your language on the next time you will see each other. What will you do in the morning? What is happening the next day? Meanwhile, reassure them that they are safe in their bed until that time. Validate their feelings, while keeping your boundaries.

Camping out

Camping out is a gentle sleep training technique that gradually reduces parental presence. To camp out, start by sitting near your child's bed at bedtime, providing verbal reassurance but avoiding excessive engagement or physical touch. Over several nights, move the chair farther away (for example, from bedside to the middle of the room, then to the doorway, then out of sight). Eventually, reassure the child from outside the room, checking in at longer intervals until they fall asleep independently.

For some kids, camping out starts by staying in their room the entire night. Use an inflatable mattress or sleeping bag for yourself so that you aren't lying in their bed. If they wake in the night, they will gain immediate reassurance of your presence, avoiding the stress hormone rise. Over time, move your mattress farther away from the bed until you are outside the room and they are sleeping through the night.

WARNING

Beware the extinction effect! It's not uncommon for you to see a *regression* in sleep behaviors a few days after initiating a sleep training method. This normal reaction occurs because your child is beginning to understand that *your* behavior has changed around bedtime, often causing an increase in the intensity of the protests. If your child starts to demonstrate an extinction burst, understand that this is a temporary and necessary part of the process. Hold firm to your plan, and keep pressing on.

Scheduling check-ins

For this method, you preempt anxiety-driven wake-ups by checking in at predictable intervals *before* your child starts calling out (for example, every 5–10 minutes at first, then increasing time gaps). Scheduled check-ins reduce separation distress, reinforcing your return without their need to get your attention.

TIP

Be sure to do your check-ins at expected time intervals. A common mistake is not to do the check-in because your child seems okay. Remember, kids are tricky and may be testing your follow-through by pretending to be asleep. If this happens, it undermines the trust you are trying to build.

CIRCADIAN SCIENCE

Melatonin, a hormone primarily produced by the pineal gland, regulates the sleep-wake cycle. Secretion patterns of this hormone undergo significant developmental changes from infancy through adolescence. Patterns are influenced by age, environmental light exposure, and circadian system maturation.

During early childhood, melatonin production typically begins between 6:00 and 8:00 p.m., contributing to a strong evening sleep drive. Melatonin levels are higher in early childhood than in later years, supporting earlier bedtimes. As children age, melatonin onset shifts and secretion duration shortens, leading to later bedtimes and reduced sleep duration. Exposure to screens emitting blue light can further suppress melatonin production, affecting sleep patterns.

Understanding melatonin onset and its age-related changes is critical for optimizing sleep health in children and adolescents. Supplementation of melatonin at appropriate times can help to regulate a circadian rhythm. Talk with your doctor to see what they suggest.

Supplementing Sleep

It only takes one quick Amazon search for "child sleep supplements" to find hundreds of powders, liquids, and gummies promising long hours of childhood slumber. Later that day, you'll see even more ads for these popular sleep supplements in your social media feeds and inbox, backed by guaranteed promises of bedtime success. (Funny how that works.)

Do any of these supplements really help children sleep? And are they safe? You can find answers in the following sections and in Chapter 11.

Melatonin

Melatonin is a naturally occurring hormone that drives the circadian rhythm. It's the big kid on the block when it comes to sleep supplements, with nearly 1 in 5 parents offering the hormone to their children. Supplementing with melatonin is thought to increase the amount of natural hormone in your child's body and modify sleep patterns. See the nearby sidebar "Circadian science" for more information.

Despite its immense popularity and aggressive marketing, studies looking at melatonin sleep benefits have shown only modest short-term effects. Supplementation may slightly reduce sleep onset but doesn't seem to significantly increase sleep duration. Stronger support for using melatonin is seen in kids with autism spectrum disorder (ASD) and attention-deficit/hyperactivity disorder (ADHD).

Short-term use (less than 12 weeks) of melatonin is generally considered safe, but long-term studies aren't conclusive. It's sold as a dietary supplement, which can lead to variability in the consistency and quality of the product you purchase (see Chapter 11). You'll also find melatonin as an active ingredient in many combination sleep aid products.

Side effects of melatonin include nighttime waking, daytime fatigue, and vivid dreams. If you choose to try melatonin for your child, use the minimally effective dose. And avoid this supplement for kids younger than age 3 unless recommended by your prescriber.

Most parents give melatonin too close to bedtime. The optimal time to offer melatonin is a few hours before it's time to go to sleep.

Iron

Iron is an essential mineral that plays a crucial role in dopamine synthesis, a neurotransmitter required for regulating movement and arousal during sleep. There is emerging evidence of a connection between iron levels and sleep disturbances in children, particularly conditions like restless sleep disorder (RSD) and restless legs syndrome (RLS).

Before starting iron supplementation, blood levels are commonly checked. If a deficiency is found, oral replacement therapy is recommended. Dosage and administration can be determined by your pediatrician.

Magnesium

Magnesium is an essential mineral commonly associated with anxiety symptom reduction, especially in kids with ADHD. Supplementing with magnesium has also been shown to mildly improve insomnia and RLS.

Magnesium is available in various forms (see Chapter 11) and is generally well tolerated. The most common side effects are stomach upset and diarrhea. Talk to your doctor about the formulation and dosage they suggest.

Your child may already be getting enough magnesium in their diet. For foods containing magnesium see Chapter 13.

L-theanine

L-theanine is an amino acid commonly found in green tea. Recently, L-theanine has increased in popularity for the treatment of insomnia in children, especially those with ADHD. It's thought to promote relaxation by boosting levels of GABA and serotonin and lowering levels of excitatory hormones.

L-theanine is generally considered safe and is recognized by the U.S. Food and Drug Administration (FDA). Although commonly found in multi-ingredient sleep supplements for kids, an optimal or effective dosage for children is not known. Talk to your doctor to find out more.

Examining Anxiety in Toddlers

Toddler brains are just starting to build social-emotional skills. From years 1–3, the emotional brain is growing rapidly, including the *amygdala,* the part of the brain responsible for sensing emotion. This development allows toddlers to begin showing self-conscious emotions by 18 months, like responding with joy when someone claps for them. By 30 months, toddlers are able to exaggerate or minimize emotions based on social cues. And by age 3, they are able to cooperate, share, and control aggression.

Early development is dominated by emotion. During toddlerhood, young brains are constantly trying to make connections between the emotional brain and the thinking brain. Meanwhile, these kids are trying to navigate their world with new, incomplete, and underdeveloped pathways. When they feel threatened, it's hard for them to use these connections, leading to relative emotion brain dominance.

REMEMBER

Being anxious is a normal part of life. It's when unreasonable fears and worries start to dominate thinking and change behaviors that anxiety becomes abnormal.

Understanding toddler fears

Toddlers have a keen sense of self-preservation and vulnerability, and they interpret many things as threats — both real and imaginary. They associate certain common situations with danger, like when Mom leaves for work or when shadows look like monsters. Even when they discover that Mom comes back and the monsters turned out to be just trees, it takes repeated experiences over time for the association with danger to change.

The toddler years are when kids begin to spend more time away from their parents. They visit relatives, start preschool, and begin early social activities. Of course, this dramatic shift from being the focus of parental attention to having periods of time away from this connection, can be perceived as a threat to their safety. In addition, increased expectations for independent skills like toileting and sleeping can ramp up anxious behaviors.

REMEMBER

Young kids and toddlers *show* their emotions. Anxious behaviors include tantrums, crying, anger, avoidance, aggression, or freezing in place. They don't have the language to explain how they feel, and they're still developing the emotional regulation skills to control their response.

Remembering your role

During early emotional development, you act as an external rational brain for your young child, especially during the toddler years. In Chapter 2, I explain *social referencing,* or when a toddler turns to you to either confirm or diffuse their emotions. Social referencing is one important way to help toddlers translate the world. Let me give you an example from my office.

Michael is an active, healthy 18-month-old. He's at the office for a routine checkup. As the doctor approaches, he clings to Mom and starts to cry. At this point, his parent responds in one of two ways. Which do you think is best?

>> Michael's mom keeps a steady, warm tone and holds him securely while allowing the exam to proceed. She says, "Oh, buddy, I know the doctor seems new, but she's here to help you. Let's listen to your heart — ba-boom, ba-boom! Can you hear it?"

>> Michael's mom instantly responds with a high-pitched, rapid voice, saying, "Oh no, sweetheart. It's okay, it's okay! You don't have to be scared! I know you don't like it, and the table is too cold! But the doctor is a friend." Meanwhile, she scoops him up off the table and gives him a hug.

The first response helps Michael recognize that his uncertainty is natural but manageable, reinforcing trust and resilience. The second response, although well-intentioned, signals to Michael that his fear is justified and expected, making future doctor visits more challenging.

Taming toddler anxiety

TIP

Anxiety during toddlerhood represents healthy development of brain parts responsible for protecting them from danger. For most toddlers, these anxious moments are quickly resolved with caregiver support. The following tips may help:

>> **Practice separation.** Even when you're home, you can practice "being away." When your child is calmly playing, choose a key phrase that will trigger your leaving, like "Daddy's leaving, and I'll be back soon. I love you!" Then, go into the bathroom or around the corner for a few seconds. Announce your "return" with "Hi, I'm happy to see you" and give a hug. Consistent verbal cuing helps them to frame the cause and effect of your leaving and your return.

>> **Keep your routines.** All kids benefit from routine, but toddlers thrive with them. Add predictable sequences of events to various parts of their day to offer some tangible time stamps. Great bedtime routines (see Chapter 13) are especially important. Meal and nap times should have reproducible sequences as well.

>> **Prepare for bedtime scaries.** When imaginative thinking dominates brain pathways, it's easy to misinterpret safe things for scary ones, especially in the dark. Even during times of nighttime anxiety, stick to your routines. Prolonging goodbyes and continuing to return to their room are accommodation behaviors.

>> **Don't encourage tantrums.** This one can be tricky. Of course, you don't want to ignore distress, but you also don't want to reinforce a tantrum as appropriate behavior. Name the feeling. Validate it. Wait. Reconnect when the tantrum is over. For more details on tantrums see Chapter 15.

For most kids, tantrums become attention-seeking events. Without an audience, a tantrum's power is taken away.

>> **Experiment with different coping tools.** You're figuring out how to deal with your child's emotions, as much as they are figuring out how to experience them. Dealing with anxiety and worry is a work in progress until you discover the way your unique child needs to be supported. Coping skills (see Chapter 16) can be helpful.

Watching out for concerning signs

Anxiety is pervasive thoughts of worry and fear. If your toddler's fears are so dominant that worries interfere with their daily life, or if your support isn't offering relief, it's time to reach out for help. For example, it's normal for young kids to be fearful of getting a shot at the doctor's office. However, it's not normal if the knowledge of getting a shot is so overwhelming that they are unable to stop talking about it at dinnertime, having trouble getting into the car for school because they are scared they are going to the doctor's office, or are unable to be comforted with your support.

Changing Bodies and Anxiety

Puberty is the herald of adolescence. During these years, there are drastic changes in hormone levels and a cascade of physical changes in the body and the brain. Pubertal changes like increased body hair and acne commonly begin in boys between the ages of 9 and 14 years. Girls begin puberty a bit earlier, anywhere from ages 7 to 13, with the first signs being breast changes and starting to grow taller.

REMEMBER

Pubertal development is unique in timing but consistent in its sequence. Health maintenance visits with your child's pediatrician allow routine monitoring of this process, ensuring that your child is growing optimally.

Adolescence is known to be a developmental period that carries a higher risk of anxiety. This increased risk is thought to be associated with physical changes in the brain's chemistry, along with dynamic changes in social and emotional functioning. Specifically, it's pubertal timing — not pubertal stage — that is associated with the development and severity of adolescent mental health issues, with early puberty onset carrying a greater risk.

Notably, early puberty transitions seem to be more significant for girls. Boys experience less of an impact on early body changes in a society that values size and strength. However, with increased testosterone comes increased aggression that they may have difficulty controlling.

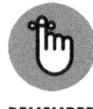

REMEMBER

If you think your child is experiencing pubertal changes too early, visit with your child's pediatrician. They can perform a physical exam and look at growth rates to determine whether your child is growing too early or too quickly. If there are concerns, your doctor will refer your child to a pediatric endocrinologist, a doctor who specializes in puberty changes and hormones, for additional testing and evaluation.

When kids start puberty, most parents expect a certain level of behavioral changes. Puberty brings a change in attitude, with kids often drawing closer to peers and away from parental companionship. Kids in adolescence pay more attention to how they look and dress, caring more about what their peers think of them. Moods and emotions are expected to shift, with changes in behavior like spending more time in their rooms or less time doing the things they used to enjoy with the family.

REMEMBER

These changes to your child's attitude and behavior can seem abrupt, and sometimes severe. It can be very hard to tell whether the changes you're seeing are normal or signs of a more significant problem. The following are some things to consider when determining if your adolescent may need help:

» **Does your child have at least one good friend?** Kids don't need a large group of friends to get through puberty. The quality of friendships plays a more crucial role than the quantity. High-quality friendships provide essential support during times of stress, boost confidence, and improve decision-making abilities. Fostering and maintaining even a small number of meaningful friendships is key to building resilience in children. If your child is pulling away from peers and choosing to isolate themselves, it's a cause for concern.

» **Does your child have at least one adult they can talk to?** Research indicates that the presence of at least one stable, supportive adult relationship is crucial for fostering resilience in children. These relationships can buffer children from developmental disruptions and help them develop the skills needed to adapt to adversity. Although having multiple supportive adults can provide additional benefits, the key factor is ensuring that every child has at least one such relationship to promote healthy development.

» **Does your child have at least one activity that engages them and brings them joy?** This can be a sport, music, school subject, or anything that involves learning and developing a skill set. Participating in hobbies and leisure activity decreases stress hormones and elevates mood. Hobbies in a social setting also offer opportunities for connection and belonging.

» **Does your child have some good, happy days?** It's normal for preteens to have more general irritability and show annoyance. Some may have more aggression and anger. But in between these moments of distress, you should be able to see some days with recognizable joy and happiness. If your child is consistently down, disengaged, or discontent, it's time to reach out for help.

» **Does your child engage in self-harm or self-sabotage?** This can include physical harm to themselves, but also things like using alcohol or drugs, choosing to skip school, or breaking laws. It's normal to be curious about these things, but you should be seeking help if you think your child's health or well-being is being threatened by these types of activities.

Co-Parenting an Anxious Child

Kids with anxiety live in all types of families. The ability of separated families to raise well-adjusted, healthy, and happy kids is equal to that of intact families. However, separated families have unique challenges for children with anxiety, especially when differences in parenting philosophies or lack of predictability exists.

Focusing on your child

I appreciate and have witnessed how brutally painful separation can be for families. When nothing can be done to restore something broken, the feelings of sadness, helplessness, and pain can be overwhelming. Your reaction to the separation heavily influences your child's experience. Be sure that you're supporting yourself through the process using healthy coping skills, like taking time for self-care, connecting with friends and support groups, and leaning into professional help as you need.

REMEMBER

Connections to supportive and loving parents mitigate the negative effects of stress. For every co-parenting decision, ask how the decision will support the health and wellness of your child. As challenging as it can be, try to compromise. Co-parenting is not about winning or losing; it's about creating nurturing spaces, continuing connection, and putting the love for your child first.

Informing and communicating

Effective communication supports co-parenting collaboration. Shared calendars, brief check-ins, or more formal family meetings are ways to avoid confusion and ensure a shared journey. In addition, communication allows co-parents to reach common goals and create stable routines.

Anxious kids need predictability. Whether it's living arrangements, transitions, vacations, or holiday plans, find common ground with your co-parent where possible, and be flexible enough to compromise when you can't. Share these plans with your child so that they know what they can expect.

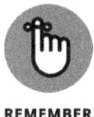

Anxiety is about avoidance. Kids can play off each co-parent to avoid stressful situations or environments, like begging to stay with Mom at drop-off or refusing to pack up their things for a pick-up. Consistent communication can help to identify avoidance behaviors and mitigate their continuation.

Handling drop-offs and pick-ups

Living in separate homes comes with necessary transitions, often drop-offs and pick-ups, when a child leaves one co-parent for the other. Successful transitions have elements of routine and support, but they are influenced by your child's innate temperament and feelings of attachment. Experimenting with different elements of co-parenting transitions can help to determine the best way your child with anxiety can cope.

TIP

When deciding on a transition plan, keep a few things in mind:

>> **Choose the best day of the week and time of day.** The day the transition takes place may influence its success. For example, it may be easier for your child to transition on Sunday after brunch than on Friday afternoon after a stressful day at school. In addition, transitioning may be easier in the morning for some kids, or the evening for others. Based on your child's experience, experiment with various times to see what may work best.

>> **Transitions are a routine.** Use routine-building techniques (see Chapter 13) to make the transition expected and predictable. Offer specific details on when the next transition will take place. Add a specific, recognizable ritual to look forward to.

>> **Model kindness.** Be confident and polite to your co-parent.

>> **Keep it brief.** Prolonging transitions is an accommodation behavior that can make anxiety worse.

Parenting in your own home

You can only control what happens in your own home. It's hard not to get upset or resentful if your child's other parent is not doing something that you feel is important. But as difficult as it is to see inconsistencies, successful co-parents allow variability. What happens in each home, outside of frank neglect or abuse, belongs to each parent. And each parent deserves respect and autonomy to experiment with their own strengths to find ways to support their child.

Feel confident in your choices. Not uncommonly, kids will get upset when "Mom doesn't make me do that at her house." This reaction is normal, especially if an "ask" challenges an existing fear association. Respond calmly. Explain that each parent can do different things and that's okay. Offer connection and validation, but continue to expect your child to follow through.

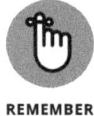

REMEMBER

Kids are amazingly adaptable to a variety of supportive environments. Focus your efforts on making your home and behaviors as supportive as you can. You may be able to communicate techniques that have worked well in your environment to your co-parent, but even if they choose to try it themselves, it may not work in a different place. Some things are impossible to duplicate, and more than one thing often works.

5

The Part of Tens

Understand that needle or "shot" phobia is common in young children. Introduce ways to support a child through medical injections of all types.

Know the signs to watch for that signal a child's need for professional help.

Find helpful and supportive phrases every parent should keep in their back pocket to encourage problem-solving, discourage avoidance, and show empathy.

Turn to useful resources for parents of kids with anxiety, including plenty of books and websites, in the Appendix.

Chapter **18**

Ten Ways to Support Kids Who Fear Needles

Most kids are nervous about needles. Let's face it — no one loves getting a poke. However, kids will experience needles as part of growing up. Routine vaccinations, IV insertions, and getting stitches are normal life experiences during childhood. Making the experience as comfortable as possible is the goal.

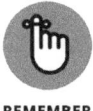

REMEMBER

Your job as a parent isn't to remove all the difficult and painful experiences from your child's path. Your job is to provide support and love through those moments.

Needle phobia is directly associated with long-term health. Adults with needle phobia are more likely to delay, skip, or defer routine preventative care for themselves *and their children*, potentially increasing the risk of missing early signs of disease.

Adults with needle phobia have lower vaccination rates, directly increasing their risk of preventative disease. Finally, parents with needle phobia may unintentionally transfer their anxiety to their kids, making child healthcare appointments more stressful and challenging.

If your child is nervous about needles, it's okay. Your child is neither unique nor alone. Here are ten ways to help support a needle-fearing child before, during, and after the appointment.

Preparing Your Child in Advance

Based on your child's temperament, choose when to explain they will be getting an injection. Some kids want to know the day before to mentally prepare. Other kids need to know the day of, when they arrive to the office, or don't need to know in advance at all.

TIP

For kids who are especially fearful about needles, "surprising" them with an injection is not ideal. This conditions them to be more anxious every time they walk into the doctor's office because they are never sure what will happen. Be sure to give anxious kids appropriate notice that an injection is coming.

TIP

Young kids learn and prepare through play. Find a storybook that walks through a doctor visit and injections. Read the story and play along with a pretend doctor kit. At the office, repeat the same phrasing as the book character. This will help your child associate the experience that the character was able to successfully complete with their real-life event.

For older kids, ask whether they have any questions about the injection. Be open to hearing their feelings and offer any explanations. Do they have a question you can't answer? Great! I love to know that my older patients are thinking about what's happening to their body. Have your kid bring their questions to the visit so the doctor can have an opportunity to explain.

Never promise "no shots." If you aren't sure whether a child will get an injection, say you don't know. The no-shot promise is a subtle, but powerful, accommodation behavior that can make the actual experience of getting an injection more anxiety-provoking and painful. If your child really needs to know whether injections will be given during the office visit, call the office before you arrive to confirm the plan.

Explaining Needles in Simple Terms

Young kids need honest and simple explanations about needles. Use age-appropriate language in a positive manner to describe the needle experience. For younger kids, you may try one of the following phrases:

>> "You are getting a tiny pinch in your arm to help keep you healthy. It will be over fast, and I'm going to be with you the whole time."

>> "The nurse is going to give you a special medicine to help your body feel better. It may feel like a little sting, but it's just for a second, and then you will be all done."

>> "It's okay to be nervous, but the nurse is the best! Once you're done, we can go to the park."

Older kids tend to have more curiosity about what exactly is being done with the needle. Typically, they already understand that needles are uncomfortable and quick. Support older kids by reinforcing this message honestly, while adding context:

>> "The nurse uses a needle to take a small amount of blood from your arm. Then it goes to the lab and gets looked at under the microscope. This helps tell the doctor why you have been feeling tired. Once we know more, we can get you feeling better."

>> "An immunization gives your body instructions on how to fight against a disease. This is important to keep your body healthy and protected."

>> "Injections aren't fun, but they are an important way to keep your body safe and healthy. It's normal to be nervous, but you are being brave and taking care of your health. That's awesome."

Modeling Calmness

Your kids look to you for emotional cues. If you're nervous about something, they may mimic that energy. Projecting calmness can help diffuse your child's worry. Being calm when your child is going to get an injection isn't always easy, but you have the ability to control your emotions better than your child.

Model calmness in your words, expression, and body language. Speak slowly and in a positive tone. Keep explanations brief and factual, focusing on the feeling of pride when the injection is over. Keep your body language open and relaxed. If helpful, sit near them or hold their hand. Reinforce positive behaviors your child uses to relax. Finally, model self-compassion. Acknowledge any stress and demonstrate how you are getting through it.

Advocating for Pain Management

Evidence-based pain management techniques should be used during all medical procedures. These vary from simple distraction techniques to using medications to decrease the discomfort. Pain is best relieved when multiple pain-reducing strategies are used. Here are ways to help:

>> Applying topical anesthetic cream is an easy and relatively inexpensive way to reduce injection pain. Lidocaine cream is available without a prescription.

TIP

Be sure to apply a thick layer of the anesthetic cream to the proper injection site. This may be in the inner arm for a blood draw or the upper outer arm for a vaccination. If you aren't sure of the location, call your doctor. Cover the cream with plastic wrap to keep it in place. The cream needs to be applied at least 1 hour beforehand for best effect. You may notice a slight paleness of the skin when the medication begins to take effect.

>> Using additional tools for pain reduction, like ice packs, cooling spray, or pain-blocking devices, is also common in many pediatric offices. Ask your provider about options they have available.

>> Choosing a comfortable position for your child during the procedure is also helpful. If it's safe, avoid lying your child on their back. Rather, keep your child sitting up on the exam table, in your lap, or near you in a chair. Stay close to your child to hold hands or provide physical comfort.

Allowing Control Where Possible

During medical procedures, anxiety increases due to the feeling of lack of control. In some kids, this can lead to aggressive behaviors, rage, or anger. To avoid this, engage your child in decision-making when they can. The following list is a few examples of options that may be available:

>> Do you want the injection in your right or left arm?

>> Would you like to sit in the chair or on the exam table?

>> After the injection, do you want a sticker or a toy?

>> Which Band-Aid would you like after the procedure is over?

>> Do you want to listen to music or watch a cartoon?

REMEMBER

Your child doesn't get a choice about whether they get an injection. Excusing a child from getting a shot is an unhelpful accommodation behavior that allows them to avoid fear.

Getting the Injection First

During most office visits, the doctor visits with the family before any injections are given. For kids with needle phobia, the anticipation of getting the injection increases their fear. Meanwhile, the kids aren't able to fully participate in the visit because they are only worrying about what comes next.

For kids with needle fear, I encourage families to get the injections during the first part of the visit. This allows the child to relax for the remainder of the visit, improves communication with the doctor, and lessens everyone's anxiety in the room. If getting injections first sounds like it may be helpful for your child, talk with your doctor's office before you arrive to arrange the plan.

Engaging in Distraction

Distraction is a strategy to take your child's attention away from the procedure at hand. You can distract your child during the injection with physical items like toys, simple games, or screen time. Help your child pay attention to the distraction item being used by playing with them or asking about what they are watching.

You can also successfully distract your child by talking about non-procedure-related topics, like stories, humor, or a favorite activity. Stay focused on your child to keep their attention on the conversation.

TIP

Apologizing or providing excessive reassurance has been shown to increase a child's anxiety and pain. Choose your words mindfully to avoid these verbal traps.

Practicing Breathing Techniques

Kids over the age of 3 can be coached to take deep, slow breaths for pain reduction. Model this type of breathing before and during the injection so your child can follow along. For more on breathing techniques for anxiety reduction see Chapter 16. Be sure to stay calm and confident while using these techniques with your child.

Celebrating the Accomplishment

Overcoming fear is something to be celebrated. After the injection is over, it's time to offer a special treat. This can be a favorite event, small prize, or fun snack. Keep the reward simple and appropriate to the accomplishment.

While you're celebrating, take a minute to review the day. Remind your child how their choices and behavior shaped their experience, and explain the health benefits of the procedure. Reinforce confidence in the successful techniques and explain how they can continue to use them in the future.

Seeking Professional Help

For children with needle phobia, the fear of any procedure using a needle significantly interferes with their ability to get proper medical care. These kids worry about every doctor visit, have extreme emotional and physical responses to injections in the office, and attempt various avoidance behaviors to steer clear of needles.

REMEMBER

Like other common phobias, needle phobia is a treatable condition. Various methods are used, including exposure therapy, cognitive behavioral therapy, and medications. Connecting with a mental health professional is one way to determine the most successful treatment path for your child.

Chapter **19**

Ten Signs Your Child Needs Professional Help

R esearch clearly shows that evidence-supported therapies can prevent early emotional struggles from becoming long-term disorders. For the kids who need it, getting help really works, and it's too important to miss. This chapter highlights ten signs to watch out for in your anxious child.

REMEMBER

If your child expresses suicidal thoughts, take immediate action. Suicidal ideation is a medical emergency, and delaying care could lead to serious harm. Contact a healthcare professional or crisis line right away, such as the National Suicide Prevention Lifeline (988). If your child is in immediate danger, call 911 or go to the nearest emergency room.

Avoiding Things They Love

One foundation of childhood is joyful play. Lots of it. From babies to big kids, all children need to find hobbies and activities that bring them joy, friendships, and fun. Although the activities themselves may change over time, the desire to play should remain. When children choose to pull away from the things they formerly enjoyed, it's a red flag for trouble.

Regressing Behaviors

Every person deals with stress differently, including our kids. During times of life transition, like welcoming a new baby or moving to a new home, behavior changes for a few weeks are typical and expected. Consistency and emotional support will get most kids back on track.

If undesired or concerning behaviors last a month or more, it's time to talk with your child's doctor to see whether more support is needed. For kids with anxiety, concerning behaviors include unexplained tantrums, aggression, sleep changes, clinginess, and more.

Missing School

School is a child's work, and kids need to be there. Persistent school avoidance is a sign of anxiety in kids, and absenteeism has a durable impact on academic performance and social progress. If your child is missing school, it's crucial to investigate underlying causes and seek out professional help. You can find more details about school avoidance in Chapter 14.

Displaying Physical Symptoms

Mood disorders affect the whole body, not just the brain. As I discuss in Chapter 4, physical manifestations are one part of child anxiety. As anxiety escalates and persists, so do the physical symptoms. Any persisting physical symptoms need to be thoroughly evaluated by a medical professional, especially if the symptoms align with known stressors or have a significant impact on your child's daily functioning.

Disrupting the Family

When parents describe their child behaviors as making the family "walk on eggshells," it's a red flag for help. Anxious kids with significant and rapid mood changes, aggressive behavior, and persisting defiance cause whole-family disruption. Choosing to pursue professional help can relieve family stress and improve parent-child relationships.

Dropping Academic Marks

Anxiety interferes with a child's ability to focus in school or complete homework due to racing thoughts and excessive worry. If your child is going to school but their performance is dropping, investigation is warranted.

TIP

Keep in mind that the neurotransmitters and brain parts involved in anxiety overlap with various other conditions, including attention-deficit/hyperactivity disorder (ADHD) and learning disabilities. These types of issues can only be supported when correctly identified by a professional.

Engaging in Self-Destructive Behaviors

REMEMBER

Behaviors that cause physical or emotional harm to oneself can indicate mood disorders and require professional help. Young kids may hit themselves, bang their heads, or engage in dangerous activities like running into traffic or jumping from high places. Older kids may start harmful self-criticism or self-sabotaging friendships. At any age, if a child is harming themselves through cutting, scratching, or bruising, they need a professional evaluation.

Choosing Isolation

Young kids prefer to hang around their family, especially before the teen years. So if your child starts pulling themselves away from family activities, spending large amounts of time in their room, or skipping group events, take it as a possible sign that something is wrong.

Asking for Help

There has been an increase in mental health awareness at all education levels. For example, in many areas of the country, kids as young as kindergarten are learning emotional literacy from school counselors and are aware that there are people who can help kids with feelings. That being said, if a child ever asks you directly for mental health help, make an appointment with your pediatrician or mental health clinician. They will have the expertise and communication skills required to dig deeper into your child's emotional state and ensure that they are safe.

Receiving Encouragement from Professionals

We all know it takes a village. Your kids will interact with many trusted adults throughout their life. Teachers, doctors, coaches, tutors — these are people who have a vested interest in the health and wellness of all the children they care for. If another adult or professional reaches out and expresses concern about your child's mental health, take it seriously.

REMEMBER

Getting professional help is not a weakness, a character flaw, or a reflection on your parenting. For kids with anxiety, medical and therapeutic support is effective, evidence-supported, and potentially lifesaving. If you just can't shake a worry about your child's mental health, or you notice concerning behavior changes, reach out for help. Medical and mental health professions are here to support your entire family and get the help your child needs.

Chapter **20**

Ten Things to Say to Your Anxious Child

S upporting a child with anxiety takes all of you: body language, facial expressions, physical touch, eye contact, and your voice. Learning a few supportive phrases is one way to prepare for times your child is getting overwhelmed and stressed.

TIP

Committing these ten phrases to memory isn't a bad idea. Within them, you'll find the words you need to support your anxious child in nearly any situation. *Hint:* The last one is the most important.

"I'm Here with You, and We'll Get Through This Together."

This powerful phrase helps kids know that they aren't alone in their struggle. To a young child, anxiety can feel very isolating, bizarre, and scary. They don't know why their brain is working the way that it is, and they don't know how to change its messages on their own. By using these words, you reflect reassurance and comfort through their feelings of isolation or helplessness. Using this phrase also promotes relationship and safety.

"It's Okay to Feel Scared or Worried Sometimes."

This is a phrase of validation. Validation is a form of empathy. It lets your child know that experiencing anxiety is a normal part of being human, allowing them to accept their feelings even when it's uncomfortable. When children feel their emotions are heard and respected, they're more receptive to learning coping strategies and gradually facing fears.

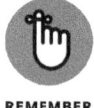

REMEMBER

When you validate a child's anxiety, it doesn't mean you're agreeing with or reinforcing anxious behaviors — you're simply acknowledging your child's emotional experience as real and legitimate. This is an important distinction.

"Is This a Big Problem or Small Problem?"

Anxiety makes kids exaggerate risk and catastrophize. This question helps them pause, reassess, and gain perspective. In turn, they gain a sense of control. This approach helps to differentiate urgent from non-urgent issues, build confidence, and reinforce the idea that challenges can be faced rather than feared.

"Let's Take Slow, Deep Breaths Together."

This phrase encourages co-regulation, or the action step you can take to demonstrate a calming technique. When your young child is anxious, they rely on your steady presence to feel safe and regulate their emotions. Over time, as they observe and practice calming techniques, they learn to self-regulate and manage anxiety on their own.

"What's Making You Feel Anxious Right Now?"

This open-ended phrase gives your child a chance to express their fears. This helps them feel seen and avoids the possibility that you may misinterpret their trigger. Especially if you have anxiety yourself, your interpretation of your child's anxieties may be heavily biased by your own worries. Allowing them to share their experience directly offers an opportunity to gather insight and develop effective problem-solving strategies to help in the future.

"This Feeling Will Pass. It May Take a Little Time, but It Will Get Better."

Anxiety creates a stress cascade that takes time to naturally fade. Meanwhile, the symptoms may make your child feel out of control. This phrase provides reassurance that the symptoms they are experiencing are not harmful to their body and will pass in time. This helps make them feel more grounded and gives them an awareness of how anxiety feels in their body.

"You're Really Strong for Facing This. I'm Proud of How You're Handling It."

Use this phrase to reinforce hard things. Kids with anxiety are asked to do the exact *opposite* of what their body and brain are telling them to do — that's really hard work. This phrase reinforces their effort, builds their self-esteem, and encourages them to try it again. As a follow-up, you can ask them what (small) next step they're going to try when they experience the situation again.

"Let's Think of Some Ways We Can Make This Situation Easier."

Part of working through anxiety is fostering a sense of agency and control. This phrase actively involves your child in this type of problem-solving work, building the foundation that's required to repeat this exercise in the future. Phrasing worries this way will all them to problem-solve on their own and prevent avoidance.

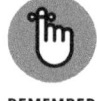

REMEMBER

Avoidance is a key feature of child anxiety, reinforcing fear by preventing your child from learning that feared situations are safe. All evidence-supported anxiety treatments focus on gradually reducing avoidance.

"You've Handled This Before, and I Know You Can Do It Again."

Anxious kids often struggle to recognize their own progress. By recalling times when they faced fears, used coping skills, and overcame challenges, you can show them they are capable of handling anxiety again. This strengthens resilience and encourages them to trust their own ability to manage difficult emotions.

"Your Feelings Matter to Me, and I Love You."

REMEMBER

This phrase provides an opportunity to validate your child's emotional experience, while reminding them that they are accepted and loved. Kids need to feel safe in order to share important feelings and emotions with you. They need to know that no matter what they share, the love you have for them remains unbroken, and they will always be cared for. Never miss an opportunity!

Appendix

Recommended Resources

Here I list additional sources that will add detail and depth to various topics in this book. Some resources offer more general information and others offer support to unique groups of children and families.

Books about Childhood Anxiety

Many of the books available on childhood anxiety take a deep dive into therapeutic techniques to try at home. I've recommended these books to my patient families over the years:

>> *Anxious Kids, Anxious Parents,* by Reid Wilson, PhD, and Lynn Lyons, LICSW (Health Communications, Inc.)

>> *Breaking Free of Child Anxiety and OCD: A Scientifically Proven Program for Parents,* by Eli R. Lebowitz, PhD (Oxford University Press)

>> *Freeing Your Child from Anxiety: Practical Strategies to Overcome Fears, Worries, and Phobias and Be Prepared for Life — From Toddlers to Teens,* by Tamar E. Chansky, PhD (Harmony Books)

>> *Helping Your Anxious Child: A Step-by-Step Guide for Parents,* by Ronald Rapee, PhD, et. al. (New Harbinger Publications)

>> *Raising Empowered Athletes: A Youth Sports Parenting Guide for Raising Happy, Brave, and Resilient Kids* by Kirsten Jones (Triumph Books)

>> *Treating Childhood and Adolescent Anxiety: A Guide for Caregivers* by Eli R. Lebowitz, PhD and Haim Omer (Wiley)

Helpful Websites about Anxiety

There are countless online sources to support families with anxious kids. Featured here are ones that reflect evidence-based education and support for families and kids.

Websites, as well as the people who create them, change all the time. Use caution when getting advice online. If something doesn't seem right or doesn't make sense, ask a trusted health-care provider for their opinion.

General information

These sites offer general information about childhood anxiety:

>> Anxiety and Depression Association of America (adaa.org/) offers resources and information to interested families.

>> Anxiety Canada (www.anxietycanada.com/) has a variety of basic anxiety information for children and adults, including free downloads to help you learn anxiety-reducing techniques.

>> Child Mind Institute (childmind.org/) provides awareness, education, and connection to mental health services in large metro areas of the United States. The site includes a variety of mental health topics, including video and social content.

>> Healthy Children (www.healthychildren.org/) is the parent-facing site of the American Academy of Pediatrics. Healthy Children provides information about popular topics around child anxiety, and great information about normal childhood development.

>> National Alliance on Mental Illness (www.nami.org/your-journey/kids-teens-and-young-adults/kids/) provides parents with information on a variety of mental health conditions.

>> Nemours KidsHealth (kidshealth.org/en/parents/emotions/) has excellent, reliable, and current articles for parents and kids alike — it's a go-to when looking for credible online health information.

Specific issues and conditions

The following websites offer information about more specific issues regarding anxiety and associated conditions:

» American Academy of Sleep Medicine (sleepeducation. org/healthy-sleep/bedtime-calculator/ offers a variety of sleep help, including videos and tip sheets.

» National Headache Foundation (headaches.org/) offers help with headache management, including links to their blog and podcast.

» School Avoidance Alliance (schoolavoidance.org/) provides education about school refusal behaviors and resources to use.

» Selective Mutism Association (www.selectivemutism. org/) connects you with education and resources on this rare condition.

» Tic Trainer (tictrainer.com/) is a free, web-based tic suppression tool.

» Tourette Association of America (tourette.org/ resources/overview/tools-for-parents/) offers information about Tourette syndrome and tic disorders.

» Understood (www.understood.org/) offers education and resources about conditions associated with anxiety, like ADHD.

Treatment

These websites offer help with childhood anxiety treatment:

» Academy of Cognitive and Behavioral Therapies (www.academyofcbt.org/) offers treatment information and connections to therapists.

» American Academy of Child and Adolescent Psychiatry (www.aacap.org/AACAP/Families_and_Youth/ Resources/CAP_Finder.aspx) includes information on medical management, including a free anxiety medication guide download and a psychiatrist finder feature.

>> Association for Behavioral and Cognitive Therapies (www.abct.org/featured-articles/childrens-mental-health/) provides information about CBT and has a therapist finder feature.

>> Baylor College of Medicine (www.bcm.edu/research/faculty-labs/luna-learning-to-understand-and-navigate-anxiety) offers free CBT modules for kids and parents through their Learning to Understand and Navigate Anxiety (LUNA) program.

>> British Association for Behavioral and Cognitive Psychotherapies (babcp.com/) is a professional organization that helps connect families to CBT therapists in the United Kingdom and Ireland.

>> Cool Little Kids (www.coollittlekids.org.au/login) offers an online course for parents of anxious children ages 3–6 years.

>> Coping Cat (www.copingcatparents.com/) has tips, support, and courses for parents of anxious children and kids ages 7 and older.

>> Society of Clinical Child and Adolescent Psychology (effectivechildtherapy.org/) offers free online assessment tools, excellent information on evidence-based therapies, and a therapist finder tool.

>> SPACE (www.spacetreatment.net/) is a parent-based treatment program. This site offers resources and connections to therapists.

>> Stanley-Brown Safety Planning Intervention (suicide safetyplan.com/forms/) provides free downloads that can be used to construct a safety plan for suicide prevention.

>> The 988 Suicide and Crisis Lifeline (988lifeline.org/) offers 24/7 connection to counselors during difficult moments.

Additional support

These sites offer additional support for families of children with anxiety:

>> Center for Parent Information and Resources (www.parentcenterhub.org/getting-started-for-families/) offers resource and webinars for families interested in education advocacy.

>> Exercise Right (exerciseright.com.au/exercise-right-kids-resources/) offers fact sheets to help all children, including those with disabilities, get safely moving every day!

>> Let Grow (letgrow.org/) offers support and connections for parents interested in encouraging independent childhood play.

>> Triple P (www.triplep-parenting.com/us/triple-p/) is the Positive Parenting Program that features information and courses that help parents increase childhood independence and resilience.

>> USP (www.usp.org/verification-services/verified-mark) and NSF (www.nsf.org/) are certification labs for various supplements and nutraceuticals, offering reference standards and other consumer-based information.

Index

B

background stressors, rise in anxiety and, 34–35

back-to-school anxiety, 224–225

Baylor College of Medicine (website), 310

B-complex vitamins, 181, 212

BEARS sleep screening, 118

bedsharing, 204–206

bedtime pass technique, 271–272

behavior contract, as a strategy for behavioral management, 245

behavior management strategies, 237, 238–252

behavioral activation, as a side effect of SSRIs, 156–157

behavioral inhibition (BI), 37

behavioral insomnia, 81

behavioral intervention therapy, 94

behaviorally inhibited (BI) temperament, 50

behaviors, 45–46, 47, 238–239

black box warning, 157

blood pressure, increased, as a side effect of SNRIs, 159

books, as resources, 307

boundaries, creating and enforcing, 243

brain
about, 18–19, 21
alpha-agonists and, 159
antihistamines and, 160
challenges in pediatric mental health, 29–30
developing, 36
emotional regulation, 24–25
fuel for the, 13
hindbrain, 19
inner, 20
neurotransmitters, 22–24
outer, 20
plasticity of, 21–22
sleep and, 202
SNRIs and, 158
social-emotional milestones, 25–29
SSRIs and, 154–155

brain-body connection, 72

bravery, 250–251

Breaking Free of Child Anxiety and OCD: A Scientifically Proven Program for Parents (Lebowitz), 307

breathing techniques, 257–258, 293

British Association for Behavioral and Cognitive Psychotherapies (website), 310

C

calming techniques
about, 207, 249, 253, 257
breath control, 257–258
cognitive engagement, 260–261
grounding, 258–260
panic attacks, 263–268
regulation, 254–255
teaching, 255–257
using, 261–262

calmness, modeling, 290

camping out, 272–273

cannabidiol (CBD), 183–184

carbohydrate malabsorption, as a cause of CAP, 76

cardiovascular system, sleep and, 202

caregivers, doctor visits and, 104

case studies, 42–43

celebrating accomplishment, for needle phobia, 293

Celexa (citalopram), 154

Center for Parent Information and Resources (website), 311

Centers for Disease Control and Prevention (CDC), 10, 32

central nervous system (CNS), 18, 74, 159

Chansky, Tamar E. (author), 307

Cheat Sheet (website), 3

check-ins, scheduling, 273

chest pain, 90–92

child development, 9–10

Child Mind Institute (website), 308

Children's Sleep Habit Questionnaire (CSHQ), 118

child-resistant packaging, 162

cholesterol, increased, as a side effect of SNRIs, 159

chronic abdominal pain (CAP), 73–80

circadian system, 273

cleanliness, urinary issues and, 89

cognitive behavioral therapy (CBT), 13, 139–140, 145

cognitive engagement, 260–261

cognitive restructuring, 139

cognitive testing, in psychological evaluations, 118–119

comfort, urinary issues and, 89

communication, 244, 282–283

community clinics, for therapy, 134

co-morbidity, 12, 122, 252

conditions, websites for, 309

confidentiality, with doctors, 106–107

confusional arousal, 81

consequences, preparing, 243–244

consistency, 248, 262

constipation, 76, 77–78, 89

context, searching for, 246–247

contributing, to anxiety, 191

Cool Little Kids (website), 310

co-parenting, 282–284

Coping Cat (website), 310

coping skills, 129, 192, 279

co-regulation, 256–257, 262

cortex, 20, 21

costs
  of supplements, 175
  of therapy, 134

Cymbalta (duloxetine), 158

D

deep breathing, for CAP, 79

defiance, 246–247

dentist, 83

depression, 50, 122–123

developmental milestones. See social-emotional milestones

developmental phases, 18

developmental skills, 241

diagnosis, 11–12, 122–124

dialectical-behavior therapy for children (DBT-C), 140

diet, 211–214

diphenhydramine, 160

disorders of gut-brain interaction (DGBIs), 74

distraction, for needle phobia, 292

dizziness, as a side effect of SSRIs, 156

docosahexaenoic acid (DHA), 177

Doctor of Philosophy (PhD), 113

Doctor of Psychology (PsyD), 113

doctors, 99, 100–110

dopamine, 24

doses, for medications, 167

drop-offs, co-parenting and, 283

dry mouth, as a side effect of SSRIs, 156

dyspepsia, as a cause of CAP, 76

E

early childhood (5-7 years), social-emotional milestones for, 27–28

early elementary school worries (age 6-8), 63

educators, doctor visits and, 103

Effexor (venlafaxine), 158

eicosapentaenoic acid (EPA), 177

electronics, urinary issues and, 89

emotional control, modeling, 233

emotional regulation, 24–25, 202

emotions, 46–47, 261

empathy, 240

enteric nervous system (ENS), 74–75, 155

environment, anxiety in children compared with adults, 51

epigenetics, 36–37

epinephrine, 23

essential nutrients, 211–212

European Medicines Agency (EMA), 171

excitatory neurotransmitters, 22

exercise, 80, 94

Exercise Right (website), 311

exhalation, 258

expectations, setting for therapy, 135–136

Eye Movement Desensitization and Reprocessing (EMDR), 141–142

F

family, 149, 203, 297

fatty acids, as an essential nutrient, 212

fears, 67–68, 69–70, 277

feedback, in psychological evaluations, 119

feelings, 46–47, 261–262

ferritin, 179–180

fiber, for constipation, 78

fight or flight response, 23, 67, 75, 263

firearms, 151–152

504 plan, 119, 226

folate, 181

follow-through phase, of therapy, 137

follow-up visits, medication and, 163

food allergies, CAP and, 79

Food and Drug Administration (FDA), 165, 171, 276

food elimination diets, CAP and, 79

Freeing Your Child from Anxiety: Practical Strategies to Overcome Fears, Worries, and Phobias and Be Prepared for Life - From Toddlers to Teens (Chansky), 307

fuel, for the brain, 13

functional CAP, 74

G

GABA, 24

gastric reflux, as a cause of CAP, 77

gastrointestinal (GI) changes, as a side effect of SSRIs, 155–156

general information websites, 308

generalized anxiety disorder (GAD), 55, 118

genetics, 36–37

goals, 135, 150, 163

grounding, 258–260

Group A streptococcal (GAS) infection, 94

growing pains, 83

gummies, 176

gut microbiome, 182

H

hat band headaches, 85

headaches, 84–87, 156

health, headaches and, 86

health insurance, 134, 149

healthcare provider, 11

Healthy Children (website), 308

heartburn, CAP and, 79

heating pad, for CAP, 80

Helping Your Anxious Child: A Step-by-Step Guide for Parents (Rapee), 307

hindbrain, 19

home environment

about, 199–200

diet and, 211–214

mental health and, 209–211

play, 219–221

routines, 221–222

screen time, 214–218

sleep and, 200–209

tics and, 93

homeostasis, 20

hormones, stress, 10

hydroxyzine, 160

hyperalgesia, 74

I

icons, explained, 3

imaginary fears, 67–68

immune function, sleep and, 202

imperfection, modeling, 249

individuality, respecting, 147

Individualized Educational Plan (IEP), 14, 103, 119, 227

Individuals with Disabilities Education Act (IDEA), 227

inflammatory bowel disease (IBD), as a cause of CAP, 77

inhibitory neurotransmitters, 22

initial diagnostic impression, 119

inner brain, 20

in-person therapy, 137

insurance companies, finding therapists from, 133

intentional bedsharing, 206

interference, screen time and, 216

internalizing behaviors, 45–46

N

N-acetylcysteine (NAC), 182

National Alliance on Mental Illness (website), 308

National Headache Foundation (website), 309

National Sanitation Foundation (NSF) certification, 175, 311

natural consequences, as a strategy for behavioral management, 246

needle anxiety, 287–293

Nemours KidsHealth (website), 308

neurodiversity, 123

neurofeedback techniques, for tics, 93

neuroplasticity, 129

neuroscience research, rise in anxiety and, 33

neurotransmitters, 22–24, 50

The 988 Suicide and Crisis Lifeline (website), 295, 310

nonprofit organizations, for therapy, 134

norepinephrine, 23

normalizing mental health, 33

nutraceuticals, 169–173. *See also* supplements

nuts and seeds, 212

O

obsessive-compulsive disorder (OCD), 123

obstructive sleep apnea (OSA), 82

office visits, preparing for to doctors, 101–106

omega-3 blends, 177–178

omega-3 polyunsaturated fatty acids (PUFAs), 177–178

Omer, Haim (author), 307

online therapy, 137

open door policy, for bedrooms, 153

oppositional defiant disorder (ODD), 12, 124

optimizing doctor appointments, 107–109

organic CAP, 73

organizing, before doctor visits, 101–103

outdoors, for mental health, 209–210

outer brain, 20

overcompensation, 110

overscheduling, avoiding, 220–221

P

pain management, 110, 290–291

pain reducers, for headaches, 87

pandemic effect, rise in anxiety and, 34

panic attacks, 263–268

panic disorder, 57

paradoxical excitation, as a side effect of antihistamines, 161

parental stress, rise in anxiety and, 35

parental technoference, 216

parent-child interaction therapy (PCIT), 141

parenting practices, 189–190

parenting style, 38, 187, 188–198

parents, 15–16, 39

partnerships, building, 147

Patient Health Questionnaire-9 (PHQ-9), 118

payment plans, for therapy, 134

Pediatric Acute-Onset Neuropsychiatric Syndrome (PANS), 94–95

Pediatric Autoimmune Neuropsychiatric Disorders Associated with Streptococcal infections (PANDAS), 94–95

pediatric mental health, challenges in, 29–30

Pediatric Mental Health Nurse Practitioner (PMHNP), 113

Pediatric Symptom Checklist (PSCI)/PSC-17, 117

pediatricians, 100–101, 133

perfectionism, 124

periodic limb movement disorder (PLMD), 82

permissive parenting, 188

personal recommendations, finding therapists from, 133

pharmaceuticals, 171

phobias, 53, 69–70

phrases, for anxiety, 301–305

physical discomfort, as a component of anxiety, 48

physical literacy, 232

physical symptoms
  chest pain, 90–92
  chronic abdominal pain (CAP), 73–80
  displaying, 297
  headaches, 84–87
  PANDAS/PANS, 94–95
  sleep symptoms, 80–83
  thyroid disorders, 95–96
  tics, 92–94
  urinary issues, 87–90
physiology, anxiety in children compared with adults, 49–50
pick-ups, co-parenting and, 283
pills, swallowing, 149–150
planned ignoring, as a strategy for behavioral management, 245
plasticity, of the brain, 21–22
play, 219–221
play therapy, 141
pollakiuria, 89
positive childhood experiences (PCEs), 121
positive reinforcement, as a strategy for behavioral management, 245
positivity, sports and, 234
post-traumatic stress disorder (PTSD), 141–142
pre-correction, as a strategy for behavioral management, 245
predicting anxiety, 35–38
prefrontal cortex (PFC), 20, 49
Preschool Anxiety Scale (PAS), 117
preschool worries (age 3-5), 63
prescribers, finding, 146
prevalence, 31–39, 41
Pristiq (desvenlafaxine), 158
private conversations, with doctors, 104–105
probiotics, 79, 181–182
problem-solving, as a strategy for behavioral management, 245
professional help, 89, 208–209, 293, 295–299
prompting, as a strategy for behavioral management, 245
protection, 13–14, 192
provisional tics, 93

Prozac (fluoxetine), 154
psychobiotics, 182
psychological evaluations
  about, 111
  academic testing, 118–119
  adverse childhood experiences (ACEs), 120–121
  alternatives to anxiety diagnosis, 122–124
  cognitive testing, 118–119
  explaining to children, 114–115
  feedback and recommendations, 119
  positive childhood experiences (PCEs), 121
  preparing for, 112–115
  selecting mental health clinicians, 112–113
  social determinants of health (SDOH), 120
  standardized rating scales, 117–118
  structured interview, 116
psychological flexibility, 140
psychotherapy, 129
puberty, 279–281
public speaking, fear of, 56
punishments, avoiding, 243–244

R

Raising Empowered Athletes: A Youth Sports Parenting Guide for Raising Happy, Brave, and Resilient Kids (Jones), 307
Rapee, Ronald (author), 307
reactive bedsharing, 204–206
reality-based fears, 67–68
real-world examples, of worry, 66
recommendations, in psychological evaluations, 118
recovery, prioritizing from sports, 232–233
regression, 272–273, 296
regulation, 254–255
Rehabilitation Act of 1973, 126
relationships, 129, 240
religious centers, finding therapists from, 133
Remember icon, 3
resources, recommended, 307–311
respecting individuality, 147
rest-and-digest response, 75

restless leg syndrome (RLS), 82, 275

restless sleep disorder (RSD), 275

risks

of bedsharing, 205–206

of suicide, 151

of supplements, 174

roles, 39, 239, 277–278

routines, 162, 207, 221–222, 278

S

safety, 14–15, 150–153, 241

saffron, 183

schedules, 208, 221–222, 273

school

about, 223

anxiety in, 224–225

back-to-school anxiety, 224–225

CAP and, 80

finding therapists from, 133

refusing to go to, 227–228

school-based resources for therapy, 134

support at, 14

School Avoidance Alliance (website), 309

school refusal (SR), 55, 227–228, 296

schools

finding therapists from, 133

school-based resources for therapy, 134

Screen for Child Anxiety RElated Disorders (SCARED),118

screen time, 34, 86, 208, 214–216, 217–218, 243

screening tools, for mental health, 117–118

searching for context, 246–247

selective mutism (SM), 54

Selective Mutism Association (website), 309

selective serotonin reuptake inhibitors (SSRIs), 154–157

self-administration, for medication, 162

self-care, prioritizing, 244

self-destructive behaviors, 298

self-regulation (SR), 254–255

self-reporting, 117

senses, five, 259–260

sensory processing disorder (SPD), 12

sensory processing issues, 124

separation, from toddlers, 278

separation anxiety disorder (SAD), 53–54

serotonin, 23, 145

serotonin syndrome (SS), as a side effect of SSRIs, 157

serotonin-norepinephrine reuptake inhibitors (SNRIs), 158–159

setting expectations for therapy, 135–136

shy bladder syndrome, 89–90

side effects

of alpha-agonists, 160

of antihistamines, 161

long-term, 166

of magnesium, 275

of melatonin, 275

of SNRIs, 158–159

of SSRIs, 156–157

sleep

about, 200–201

in anxious children, 204–205

bedsharing, 204–206

changes, as a side effect of SSRIs, 156

family and, 203

getting children to, 270–273

guidelines for, 203

healthy bedtime habits, 206–209

importance of, 201–202

issues with, 80–83

supplementing, 274–276

tics and, 93–94

for toddlers, 278

sleep terror, 82

sleep training, 270

sleepwalking, 82

social anxiety disorder (SoAD), 55–56

social determinants of health (SDOH), 120

social emotional milestones, 10

social referencing, 25, 277

social-emotional learning, 241–242

social-emotional milestones, 10, 25–26, 27–29

U

V

W

Y

Z

About the Author

Dr. Natasha Burgert is a board-certified pediatrician, National Spokesperson for the American Academy of Pediatrics, and child health advocate. A native of Nebraska, she earned her medical degree at the University of Nebraska Medical Center. She completed her pediatric residency at Cincinnati Children's Hospital Medical Center, one of the leading hospitals in the United States. Since that time, she's cared for children from birth through high school at her private practice in the Kansas City area.

In addition to clinical care, Dr. Natasha is a prolific writer and educator. In 2021, she earned a Certificate in Effective Writing for Health Care from Harvard Medical School. She maintains a popular newsletter addressing current pediatric health topics and shares evidence-based health information blended with expertise on various social media platforms. She has presented at national conferences and seminars, and her engaging and informative style has made her a favorite among various audiences. Find out more about Dr. Natasha and connect with her at KCKidsDoc.com.

Dedication

To the families who have entrusted me with the care of their children — thank you. Your willingness to share your stories, your fears, your joys, and your heartbreaks has been a profound privilege. This book carries the wisdom you've shared, the lessons you've taught me, and the deep respect I hold for each of you. I wrote this with your voices in my heart.

Author's Acknowledgments

I'm thankful for the team at Wiley, who carefully guided me through this wild first experience. Specifically, Elizabeth Stilwell, acquisitions editor, supported my vision for this book and gave a new author a chance. I'm thankful for the patience and talent of Georgette Beatty, my development editor, for her advice and clarity. Thanks to Kristie Pyles, my managing editor, who brought this book through layout and production. I also appreciate the exceptional editing work of Christy Pingleton and Dr. Maddie Summers, who made my words sing. Finally, I'm grateful to have the technical expertise of Dr. Nicole Baldwin woven into these pages.

I stand on the shoulders of countless professors, researchers, and attendings who taught me the joy and challenge of pediatric medicine. Their dedication to advancing science and passing wisdom to the next generation is why I have the best job in the world. I am indebted to their generosity and kindness.

My friends and family were the engine that allowed me to keep this work going and who gave me unyielding support and encouragement from concept to print. I'm thankful for their love, humor, and patience — and for making me a better human.

Finally, I'd like to acknowledge the contractor, design team, and maintenance staff at Round Pond Studio, where love beyond measure was embedded into the walls, and where this book was written.

Publisher's Acknowledgments

Associate Acquisitions Editor:
Elizabeth Stilwell

Senior Managing Editor:
Kristie Pyles

Development Editor:
Georgette Beatty

Copy Editor: Christine Pingleton

Technical Editor:
Nicole Baldwin, MD

Production Editor:
Magesh Elangovan

Cover Image: © Peathegee Inc/ Getty Images

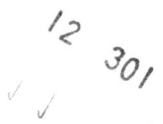